_Jackie Carson_

CLINICAL
**SKILLBUILDERS**™

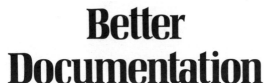

# Better Documentation

C L I N I C A L
## SKILLBUILDERS™

# Better
# Documentation

Springhouse Corporation
Springhouse, Pennsylvania

# STAFF

**Executive Director, Editorial**
Stanley Loeb

**Editorial Director**
Matthew Cahill

**Clinical Director**
Barbara F. McVan, RN

**Art Director**
John Hubbard

**Senior Editor**
William J. Kelly

**Clinical Project Editor**
Judith A. Schilling McCann, RN, BSN

**Editors**
Margaret Eckman, Kevin Law, Elizabeth Mauro

**Clinical Editors**
Lynore D. DeSilets, RN, EdD; Mary Gyetvan, RN, BSEd

**Copy Editors**
Jane V. Cray (supervisor), Nancy Papsin, Doris Weinstock

**Designers**
Stephanie Peters (associate art director), Matie Patterson (senior designer), Linda Franklin

**Illustrators**
John Gist, Robert Jackson, Robert Neumann, Judy Newhouse, Dennis Schofield

**Art Production**
Robert Perry (manager), Anna Brindisi, Donald Knauss, Thomas Robbins, Robert Wieder

**Typography**
David Kosten (director), Diane Paluba (manager), Elizabeth Bergman, Joyce Rossi Biletz, Phyllis Marron, Robin Rantz, Valerie Rosenberger

**Manufacturing**
Deborah Meiris (manager), T.A. Landis, Jennifer Suter

**Production Coordination**
Colleen M. Hayman

**Editorial Assistants**
Maree DeRosa, Beverly Lane, Mary Madden

(CCC) Transactional Reporting Service, provided that the fee of $.75 per page is paid directly to CCC, 27 Congress St., Salem, MA 01970. For those organizations that have been granted a license by CCC, a separate system of payment has been arranged. The fee code for users of the Transactional Reporting Service is 0874344093/92 $00.00 + $.75.
Printed in the United States of America.
CS9-060694

**Library of Congress Cataloging-in-Publication Data**

Better documentation.
    p.    cm. – (Clinical Skillbuilders™)
    Includes bibliographical references and index.
    1. Nursing records – Handbooks, manuals, etc.
    I. Series.    [DNLM:  1. Documentation –
    handbook.    2. Nursing Process – handbook.
3. Nursing Records – handbook.    WY 39 B5645]
RT50.B37    1992
610.73 – dc20
DNLM/DLC               91-5073
ISBN 0-87434-409-3           CIP

# CONTENTS

# ADVISORY BOARD AND CONTRIBUTORS

At the time of publication, the advisors held the following positions.

**Sandra G. Crandall, RN,C, MSN, CRNP**
Director
Center for Nursing Excellence
Newtown, Pa.

**Ellen Eggland, RN, MN**
Vice President
Healthcare Personnel, Inc.
Naples, Fla.

**Terry Matthew Foster, RN, BSN, CCRN, CEN**
Clinical Director, Nursing Administration
Mercy Hospital-Anderson
Cincinnati

**Sandra K. Goodnough-Hanneman, RN, PhD**
Critical Care Nursing Consultant
Houston

**Doris A. Millam, RN, MS, CRNI**
I.V. Therapy Clinician
Holy Family Hospital
Des Plaines, Ill.

**Deborah Panozzo Nelson, RN, MS, CCRN**
Cardiovascular Clinical Specialist
Visiting Assistant Professor
EMS Nursing Education
Purdue University, Calumet Campus
Hammond, Ind.

**Sally S. Russell, RN, MN, CS**
Instructor
Clinical Specialist
St. Elizabeth Hospital Medical Center
Lafayette, Ind.

**Marilyn Sawyer Sommers, RN, PhD, CCRN**
Assistant Professor
College of Nursing and Health
University of Cincinnati

At the time of publication, the contributors held the following positions.

**Ellen Eggland, RN, MN**
Vice President
Healthcare Personnel, Inc.
Naples, Fla.

**Mary Eileen Gribbin, RN, MSN, CNAA, ONC**
Assistant Director of Nursing
Inpatient and Ambulatory Care Division
Hospital for Joint Diseases
Orthopaedic Institute
New York

**Patricia W. Iyer, RN, MSN, CNA**
President
Patricia Iyer Associates
Stockton, N.J.

**Paula Laros Rich, RN, MSN**
Clinical Educator
Presbyterian Medical Center
of Philadelphia

**Carol Lynn Schaffer, RN, MSN, JD**
Chief Executive Officer
Cleveland Clinic Home Care
The Cleveland Clinic Foundation

In recent years, nursing documentation has become increasingly detailed and complex. For various reasons, including your own legal protection, you now must document *all* the care you give a patient. This means keeping a clear record of your assessments, writing detailed care plans, and documenting not only your interventions but also your evaluations of their effectiveness. You also need to record your patient teaching and discharge plans.

How you record much of this information will vary from one health care facility to another. But the possibilities are almost endless. Current documentation formats range from traditional narrative notes to newer innovations such as charting by exception. Plus, you may have to use some of the newer tools developed to standardize documentation, such as protocols and critical paths.

To ensure that you document the right information in the right place, you need a reliable guidebook. And that's precisely what you have in your hands. *Better Documentation,* the latest volume in the Clinical Skillbuilders series, tells you everything you need to know about documentation today. And it gives you this essential information in an easy-to-use way.

The first chapter provides an overview, covering such key concepts as the purposes of documentation, the standards your documentation must meet, and the components of the clinical record. The chapter also takes a look at the growing trend toward computerized documentation.

The next two chapters cover legal concerns. Chapter 2 explains the legal significance of the clinical record and gives you helpful guidelines on how you can chart to protect yourself and your employer. Chapter 3 discusses legal situations that call for special types of documentation — dealing with living wills, witnessing signatures on legal documents, and taking verbal orders, to name a few.

The last three chapters explain how to document the steps of the nursing process. Chapter 4 covers recording your assessments — especially your initial assessment. In Chapter 5, you'll read about how to develop nursing diagnoses, then create and document a care plan based on them. The final chapter explains how to document your nursing interventions and evaluations. In this chapter, you'll also find thorough explanations of five common documentation formats.

Throughout the book, special graphic devices called logos signal essential information about how to document. The *Timesaving tip* logo draws your attention to pointers that can save you time when you chart — how to make the most of your interview time, for example. The *Charting* logo accompanies sample documentation forms that have been filled out. Thus, you can see not only what particular forms look like but also the right way to use them. When you see a *Checklist* logo, you'll find a listing of key information. For instance, in Chapter 5, this logo signals a list of pitfalls to avoid when making nursing diagnoses.

After Chapter 6 comes a self-test that includes multiple-choice questions and a case history with an accompanying assessment form for you to fill out. Answers to the questions and a correctly completed assessment form follow.

Then, you'll find seven useful appendices. The first consists of a list of common abbreviations used on documentation forms in this book. Next, you'll find the documentation standards of the Joint Commission on Accreditation of Healthcare Organizations and the standards of practice of the American Nurses' Association. The next three appendices are helpful lists of nursing diagnoses. The first contains the diagnoses approved by the North American Nursing Diagnosis Association. Then come lists of diagnoses grouped according to the system developed by Marjory Gordon and the nursing theory developed by Dorothea Orem. The last appendix, a chart, com-

pares eight of the most important nursing theories.

With all this valuable information, *Better Documentation* will prove to be an indispensable guide. Whether you're a student or a recent graduate still learning about documentation, or an experienced nurse facing the complexities of new documentation systems, this book will serve you well. I recommend that you take it to work and use it to document with confidence.

Enea Zolezzi, RN, BSN, MHSL
Education Coordinator
Nursing Administration
California Pacific Medical Center
San Francisco

# 1

# FUNDAMENTALS OF DOCUMENTATION

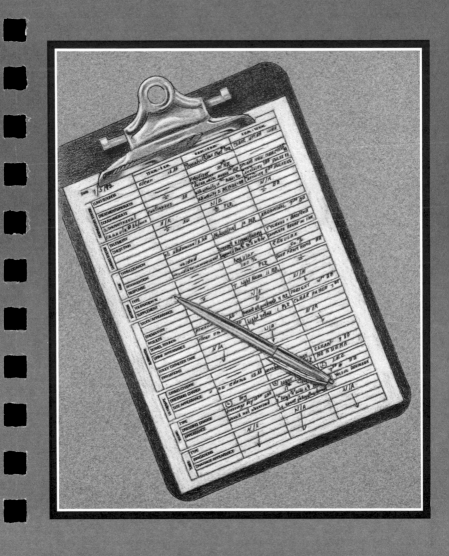

Ideally, your documentation should paint a complete picture of the care your patient receives. If you paint that picture with attention to detail, it will clearly illustrate the quality of care your patient received, the outcome of that care, and the treatment he still needs.

And such details will be scrutinized by many viewers, including other team members caring for the patient; accreditation, certification, and licensing organizations; quality assurance monitors and peer reviewers; and Medicare and insurance company reviewers. Your work may also be examined by lawyers and a judge. Or researchers and educators may use it to improve patient care and continuing education.

This chapter will give you the basic knowledge you need to create complete pictures that will satisfy these many viewers. After detailing the purposes of documentation, the chapter describes the development of the clinical record and covers the two basic types of records — source-oriented and problem-oriented. Next, you'll read about how the nursing process shapes documentation. The chapter then introduces the various formats for documenting nursing care. After that, you'll find what you need to know about the computer's impact on documentation. The chapter concludes with the documentation challenges you face today, including suggestions on how you can meet them.

# Purposes of documentation

Nursing documentation makes up one part — actually, one critical part — of the complete clinical record, which contains contributions from all health care team members. Your contribution has many purposes, including verifying the quality of your care, helping all caregivers to coordinate treatment, and providing legal protection for you and your employer.

## Quality of care
To verify the quality of your care, you must describe what you've done for your patient and provide evidence that it was necessary. You also should describe the patient's response to the care and any changes made in his care plan. Be sure to document this information in accordance with professional practice standards — those published by the American Nurses' Association (ANA) and the Joint Commission on Accreditation of Healthcare Organizations (JCAHO), for instance.

## Coordination of care
To plan interventions, make decisions about ongoing interventions, and evaluate a patient's progress, all team members need complete information on his care. And, of course, the team members rely on the clinical record for that information. So you need to ensure that your contribution is as thorough as possible.

## Accrediting and licensing
Organizations, most notably the JCAHO, accredit health care facilities that meet their standards. Some states also require all health care facilities — including home health care facilities — to become licensed. Health care facilities need JCAHO accreditation not only to demonstrate that they provide quality care, but to ensure their eligibility for government funds. The federal

government also contracts with state organizations that certify health care facilities as qualified to receive Medicare reimbursement for eligible patients.

In deciding whether a facility should receive accreditation, an accrediting organization looks at the structure and function of the facility and sometimes interviews patients. Plus, the organization always reviews the clinical record to ensure that the facility meets the required standards. Then, at regular intervals — usually annually — the organization assesses the facility for ongoing compliance. The accrediting organization conducts surveys to assess the standard and quality of care and audits the facility to ensure that it's complying with those standards.

Most accrediting organizations have some common standards for documentation. For example, most require that each patient's clinical record contain an assessment, a plan of care, medical orders, progress notes, and a discharge summary. Several organizations even spell out what these components must contain.

## Quality assurance monitoring

Mandated by state and JCAHO regulations, quality assurance activities are designed, conducted, and analyzed by designated employees of the health care facility. These employees — including administrative personnel, doctors, nurses, and pharmacists — report their findings to their Board of Trustees.

Quality assurance committees monitor, evaluate, and seek ways to improve the quality of patient care. To do this, the members of the committee develop standards, or indicators, of care. The committee members must choose well-defined,

objective, readily measurable indicators that allow them to assess the structure, process, and outcome of patient care. They can then use these indicators to monitor and evaluate the contents of the clinical record. (See *Understanding quality assurance indicators,* page 4.)

When the care described in the clinical record doesn't meet an established indicator of care, the committee decides what action to take to correct the problem. For instance, continuing education can teach employees ways to improve their care, and increased supervision or disciplinary action can correct a behavior or performance problem. And if indicators point out a structural problem, changes in institutional policy, procedure, documentation forms, or methods may improve patient care.

## Peer review

Like quality assurance committees, peer review organizations (PROs) also rely heavily on the clinical record. These PROs consist of employees who are paid by the federal government. As of 1990, nurses may serve on PROs.

Mandated by law to evaluate the quality of care provided in health care facilities, PROs evaluate a sample of a facility's clinical records and compare it with established generic screens — a list of basic conditions that a group of similar health care facilities should meet. The reviewers use these screens to determine whether the health care facility or particular caregivers provided appropriate care. For example, certain screens can help reviewers determine if personnel at a health care facility:
• minimize the risk of nosocomial infection
• maintain the medical stability of patients

## Understanding quality assurance indicators

A quality assurance indicator acts as a yardstick for assessing the clinical record—and, consequently, patient care. The quality assurance committee must develop three types of indicators: structural, process, and outcome.

### Unit and staff

Structural indicators describe the patient care environment, including the qualifications of caregivers, and help the committee assess how well a particular department functions. Structural indicators for a coronary care step-down unit might include:
• Unit has an RN-to-patient ratio of 1:4.
• All RNs on the unit have completed the hospital's coronary care continuing education program.

### Nursing actions

Process indicators focus on nursing actions. For a patient with congestive heart failure, process indicators might include:
• Assess lungs, cardiovascular status,

and peripheral pulses every shift or more often if warranted by the patient's condition.
• Obtain a daily weight.
• Assess the patient for edema, noting specific sites and the degree of edema, based on hospital protocol.
• Teach the patient or his caregiver about the medication regimen, including the adverse effects and signs and symptoms of digitalis toxicity.

### Patient outcomes

Outcome indicators focus on the results of patient care. Outcome indicators for a patient with congestive heart failure might include:
• Vital signs stay within an acceptable range, as determined by the doctor.
• Daily weight hasn't fluctuated by more than 2 lb.
• No evidence of edema exists, and intake and output are within the normal range.
• No episodes of tachycardia, bradycardia, or pulse irregularity have occurred in the last 3 days.

• minimize the need for unscheduled returns to surgery
• provide adequate discharge planning
• protect patients from avoidable trauma and death.

When a patient dies unexpectedly during or following surgery or following a return to the critical care unit within 24 hours of being transferred off of the unit, reviewers must determine if the health care facility could have prevented the death. If they find that either the facility or specific caregivers were negligent, they can discipline those at fault and suggest steps to minimize the recurrence of such incidents. If a health care facility has a higher rate of nosocomial infection

than it should, the reviewers must examine the clinical record to determine the cause.

Reviewers also look at the clinical record to determine if a health care facility truly needed to admit a particular patient and if he received the treatment that best suited his needs. Plus, PROs review complaints made by Medicare patients about care received at health care facilities. If reviewers find problems with the quality of care a patient received, they can invoke fines or sanctions, or deny reimbursement for care provided.

### Requirements for reimbursement

Documentation also helps determine the amount of reimbursement a health care facility receives. The federal government, for instance, uses a prospective payment system based on diagnosis-related groups (DRGs) to determine its Medicare reimbursements, paying a fixed amount for a particular diagnosis. For the health care facility to receive payment, the patient's clinical record at discharge must contain the correct DRG codes and verify that the patient received the correct care in the appropriate setting for the diagnoses. Your documentation should support those diagnoses and indicate that appropriate patient and family teaching and discharge planning took place.

Most insurance companies also base their payments on a prospective payment system. Typically, they won't provide reimbursement for unskilled nursing care. An examiner looks at the clinical record to determine if the patient needed and received skilled nursing care. He may even request copies of the patient's progress notes along with the monthly bills. And he'll almost certainly request progress notes to support an increase in the intensity or frequency of care because such care costs more. He'll also look for inconsistencies in documentation — for instance, a discrepancy between the treatment ordered and the treatment provided. If the examiner doesn't receive an adequate explanation for the discrepancy, the insurance company could deny payment.

### Legal protection

Good documentation should give legal protection to you, the patient's other caregivers, the health care facility, and the patient. Admissible in court as a legal document, the clinical record provides proof of the quality of care given to a patient.

Such records often serve as evidence in disability, personal injury, and mental competency cases. They're also used in malpractice cases. And what you document — or don't document — can mean the difference between winning and losing a case, not only for you, but also for your employer. For the best legal protection, make sure you not only adhere to professional standards of nursing care, but follow your employer's policy and procedures for intervention and documentation in all situations — especially high-risk situations.

### Research and continuing education

Documentation also furnishes data for research. For instance, clinical records can supply the data for a study to determine the validity of nursing diagnoses. Or a project on patient compliance may use clinical records to determine the effect of patient teaching on compliance. Such a study would probably note such variables as a patient's education level and barriers to learning, and then assess how well the patient followed the medication and treatment regimen.

These research studies can, in turn, improve documentation. For instance, a study that uncovers problems in the clinical record can point out the need for continuing education programs to make improvements.

# Clinical record

In the past, the clinical record has been referred to as the medical record. But because it consists of the contributions of all the health care team members—not just doctors—the term clinical record is growing more popular.

### Evolution of the clinical record

Decades ago, the clinical record consisted only of an admission history, a physical examination form, the doctor's orders and progress notes, laboratory and X-ray reports, and occasional narrative nurses' notes. Today, this record can include many forms, such as the initial assessment form, daily assessment flow sheets, problem or nursing diagnoses lists, and other flow sheets. Forms vary with the policies, procedures, and organizational and patient needs of individual facilities. (See *Components of the clinical record.*)

### Organization of the clinical record

Two basic methods of organizing the clinical record exist: source-oriented and problem-oriented. Each health care facility chooses one of these methods—or a variation of it—to fit its needs.

***Source-oriented narrative record.*** The traditional approach, the source-oriented narrative record requires members of each discipline—the sources—to record information in a separate section of the clinical record. Obviously, this approach makes communication among health care team members difficult. But variations of the system have alleviated this difficulty. For instance, grouping progress notes together with a different color page for each discipline allows you to determine a patient's progress more easily.

Another problem with the pure source-oriented system is its organization—or rather, lack of it. In this system, each team member writes his notes as a narrative, resulting in a clinical record that has no order of topics and often no obvious topic identification. The record has only a chronologic order—not the easiest structure for reviewing a patient's problems.

Several ways of organizing nursing documentation in the source-oriented record have been developed to make it easier to review. These include Focus charting and PIE (problem-intervention-evaluation) charting, both explained later in this chapter. But even with these variations, the basis of the source-oriented method remains the separate sources of information.

***Problem-oriented medical record.*** In 1969, Dr. Lawrence Weed of Case Western Reserve University introduced the problem-oriented medical record (POMR) as an alternative to the source-oriented record. Many health care facilities have converted, in whole or in part, to his method.

The POMR has several components:
- a compilation of baseline information
- a problem list
- an initial plan for each designated problem
- progress notes.

*Baseline information.* Taken from all disciplines, the baseline information focuses on the patient's present complaints and illnesses. It also includes social and emotional information, his medical status and history, and results of his initial physical examination and diagnostic test results. This information helps to identify the patient's problems and serves as a baseline for later assessments.

*Problem list.* Derived from the ini-

## Components of the clinical record

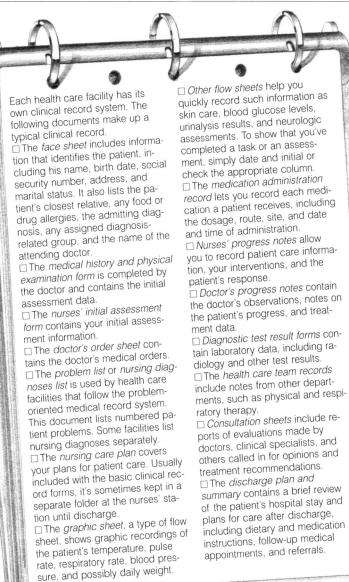

Each health care facility has its own clinical record system. The following documents make up a typical clinical record.

☐ The *face sheet* includes information that identifies the patient, including his name, birth date, social security number, address, and marital status. It also lists the patient's closest relative, any food or drug allergies, the admitting diagnosis, any assigned diagnosis-related group, and the name of the attending doctor.

☐ The *medical history and physical examination form* is completed by the doctor and contains the initial assessment data.

☐ The *nurses' initial assessment form* contains your initial assessment information.

☐ The *doctor's order sheet* contains the doctor's medical orders.

☐ The *problem list* or *nursing diagnoses list* is used by health care facilities that follow the problem-oriented medical record system. This document lists numbered patient problems. Some facilities list nursing diagnoses separately.

☐ The *nursing care plan* covers your plans for patient care. Usually included with the basic clinical record forms, it's sometimes kept in a separate folder at the nurses' station until discharge.

☐ The *graphic sheet*, a type of flow sheet, shows graphic recordings of the patient's temperature, pulse rate, respiratory rate, blood pressure, and possibly daily weight.

☐ *Other flow sheets* help you quickly record such information as skin care, blood glucose levels, urinalysis results, and neurologic assessments. To show that you've completed a task or an assessment, simply date and initial or check the appropriate column.

☐ The *medication administration record* lets you record each medication a patient receives, including the dosage, route, site, and date and time of administration.

☐ *Nurses' progress notes* allow you to record patient care information, your interventions, and the patient's response.

☐ *Doctor's progress notes* contain the doctor's observations, notes on the patient's progress, and treatment data.

☐ *Diagnostic test result forms* contain laboratory data, including radiology and other test results.

☐ The *health care team records* include notes from other departments, such as physical and respiratory therapy.

☐ *Consultation sheets* include reports of evaluations made by doctors, clinical specialists, and others called in for opinions and treatment recommendations.

☐ The *discharge plan and summary* contains a brief review of the patient's hospital stay and plans for care after discharge, including dietary and medication instructions, follow-up medical appointments, and referrals.

## Using problem lists

Below you'll find a nursing problem list for a patient with chronic obstructive pulmonary disease.

| # | Date | Problem statement | Initials | Resolved |
|---|------|-------------------|----------|----------|
| 1 | 1/4/92 | Ineffective breathing pattern related to decreased lung compliance and trapped air | J.S. | |
| 2 | 1/4/92 | Activity intolerance related to shortness of breath on exertion | J.S. | |
| 3 | 1/4/92 | Ineffective airway clearance related to copious mucoid secretions and inability to effectively expectorate mucus | J.S. | |
| 4 | 1/4/92 | Ineffective individual coping related to situational crisis | J.S. | 1/8/92 P.H. |
| 5 | 1/6/92 | Potential for infection related to alteration in kidney function | P.H. | |
| | | | | |

tial assessment data, the problem list includes both active and inactive problems and serves as an index for the entire clinical record. It's placed right at the beginning of the record to serve as a starting point for patient review, planning, intervention, and evaluation.

What qualifies as a problem can vary among health care facilities. At certain facilities, only problems that have lasted for a specific length of time, say 48 hours, may be listed. At others, only actual problems — not potential problems — may be included on the list. But however the facility defines a problem, a problem list should include acute, chronic, and (later) resolved problems in chronologic order. It can also include secondary complications, signs and symptoms, abnormal laboratory test results, and socioeconomic problems. (See *Using problem lists.*)

*Initial plan.* Based on the problem list, the initial plan for each problem should include:
• the goal of care
• plans for collecting further data, if necessary
• treatment plans
• patient education plans.

All health care team members should use these guidelines when recording entries on the initial plan. But how they use the guidelines will depend on their discipline. For instance, you might gather further data by interviewing, observing, and inspecting the patient; the doctor might do so by ordering diagnostic tests.

*Progress notes.* After you and the other team members form the initial plan, the progress notes allow you to track the changes in the patient's condition. You'll write these notes in

the SOAP (subjective, objective, assessment, and plan) format, explained more fully later in this chapter. Or you may use the SOAPIE format, adding two more categories of intervention and evaluation.

*Advantages and disadvantages.* The POMR system has several advantages, including improved communication among health care team members. Any team member can easily find the patient's problems listed at the front of the record, obtain a complete status report from a single progress note sheet, and easily find specific information in well-organized progress notes.

But the POMR system also has disadvantages. It can result in repetition — for instance, the problem list can repeat nursing diagnoses covered in SOAPIE progress notes. Plus, the SOAPIE format requires six steps to document even the simplest change in the patient's condition.

# Nursing process

Whether you document according to the source-oriented or POMR system, your documentation must reflect the nursing process. In the 1991 JCAHO accreditation manual, the updated charting guidelines reaffirm this point.

Based on theories of nursing and other disciplines, the nursing process follows the scientific method. This problem-solving process systematically organizes nursing activities to ensure the highest quality of care. It allows you to determine which problems you can help alleviate, which potential problems you

## Documentation and the nursing process

This flowchart shows the steps of the nursing process and lists the forms you should use to document them.

| Step 1: Assessment | Step 2: Nursing diagnosis |
|---|---|
| Gather data from the patient's history, physical examination, medical record, and diagnostic test results. | Make judgments based on assessment data. |
| *Documentation tools* Initial assessment form, flow sheets | *Documentation tools* Nursing care plan, protocols, critical path, progress notes, problem list |

can help prevent, what kind of and how much assistance a patient requires, who can best provide that assistance, which desired outcomes the patient can achieve, and whether the patient achieves them.

To get such a complete picture of the patient's situation, you'll need to systematically follow the five steps of the nursing process — assessment, nursing diagnosis, planning, intervention, and evaluation — and document them effectively. (See *Documentation and the nursing process.*)

### Assessment

Your assessment includes your initial general observations, the patient's history, and the physical examination as well as your ongoing observations — all of which gives you an assessment data base. You should document this data base on an initial assessment form and on flow sheets.

***Initial assessment.*** The initial assessment information you'll need and how you organize it varies with

the needs of the health care facility and, in some cases, the nursing unit. On a critical care unit, for instance, you may be required to collect information that wouldn't be necessary on a short-stay unit. To organize the initial assessment information, you may follow a body systems format. Or you may follow the new trend and use a nursing model, organizing information according to functional health patterns — sleep-rest patterns, for instance — or according to human response patterns, such as communicating. The appendices in this book provide complete lists of the functional health patterns developed by Marjory Gordon and the human response patterns developed by the North American Nursing Diagnosis Association (NANDA).

However you organize the initial assessment information, it must be complete. So make sure it covers such points as the patient's learning needs, his potential for injury, and his home care environment — including both his physical surroundings and his and the family's ability to continue vital care.

| Step 3: Planning | Step 4: Intervention | Step 5: Evaluation |
|---|---|---|
| Establish care priorities, set goals with outcome criteria and target dates, and describe interventions.<br><br>*Documentation tools*<br>Nursing care plan, protocols, critical path | Carry out planned interventions.<br><br>*Documentation tools*<br>Progress notes, flow sheets | Use objective data to assess outcome.<br><br>*Documentation tool*<br>Progress notes |

***Ongoing assessment.*** For ongoing assessment, you'll use flow sheets. A valuable assessment tool, the flow sheet provides an easy-to-read record of changes in the patient's condition over time. Originally used for fast entry of such data as intake and output and vital signs, these prepared forms have become a resource that allows all members of the health care team to easily compare data and assess the patient's progress.

Several units now use flow sheets for various purposes. Each unit may vary the flow sheet's style and format to fit its needs. In many health care facilities, assessment flow sheets are kept at the patient's bedside, serving as reminders to perform assessments and making documentation of these assessments easier. (See *Bedside documentation*, page 12.)

### Nursing diagnosis

Formulating a nursing diagnosis involves identifying actual or potential patient problems that your interventions can resolve or help resolve.

Lists of currently approved nursing diagnoses appear in the appendices.

A growing number of health care facilities use nursing diagnoses in documentation. A recent survey shows that 82% of administrators believe most of their staff members will soon use nursing diagnoses in documentation. The JCAHO approves of using nursing diagnoses in documentation, although it doesn't mandate using them.

If the policy at your facility requires that you use nursing diagnoses, you'll document them in the appropriate place in the clinical record. If the policy doesn't call for their use, you'll still need to carry out the second step in the nursing process by identifying the patient's problems and documenting them. For instance, you may record the patient's signs and symptoms or log a statement of the patient's problem, such as "Difficulty in feeding self." Depending on the policy, you may include nursing diagnoses or patient problems on the nursing care plan, progress notes, or a separate problem list.

TIMESAVING TIP

## Bedside documentation

Keeping charts at the bedside gives you immediate access to the patient's record, so you can easily record or review his care. If hospital policy allows, place the nurses' progress notes and flow sheets at the patient's bedside or outside his room on a wall-mounted chart bracket. (Such brackets commonly have an attached pull-down writing platform.)

Keep the progress notes and flow sheets at the patient's bedside for a 24-hour period. Then replace them with new forms and return the completed forms to the clinical record at the nurses' station. Keeping the rest of the clinical record at the nurses' station—the traditional centralized chart area— ensures its availability to all health care team members.

## Planning

Planning typically involves setting priorities for nursing diagnoses, identifying expected outcomes, and selecting appropriate nursing actions and target dates to achieve those outcomes.

The nursing care plan usually serves as the documentation tool for planning. It's updated as the patient's needs change or as new information suggests new or changed problems, needs, or nursing diagnoses.

Still widely used, the traditional nursing care plan calls for you to develop and write out plans for each patient's care in detail—a task that requires a good deal of time and thought. But changes in the JCAHO's requirements that allow more flexibility and the introduction of new ways of documenting are making care planning faster and

easier. Standardized nursing care plans, critical paths, and protocols may soon be used with, or take the place of, the traditional plan. All three meet quality assurance standards and can save you time.

*Standardized plans.* A preprinted care plan, each standardized nursing care plan is designed for a typical patient with a specific disorder or nursing diagnosis. To use one of these plans, you'll need to individualize it for your patient by adding and deleting information.

*Critical paths.* A critical path, or health care map, covers key interventions for a patient with a specific diagnosis and allows easy monitoring of his progress. Take a patient who has undergone abdominal surgery. The critical path may recommend that you have him progress from complete bed rest to sitting in a chair the day after surgery and that you have him try to walk in the hall 4 days after surgery.

*Protocols.* Protocols specify a sequence of actions to follow to manage a specific problem or need. They were originally used to manage equipment (such as mechanical ventilators) or a phase of hospitalization (such as preoperative care), but their use has been expanded. Many health care facilities now use them to stipulate care for patients with specific nursing diagnoses, often in combination with traditional or standardized nursing care plans or critical paths.

*Discharge plans.* No matter what type of care plan you use, you must include plans for discharging the patient. With shorter hospital stays, your patients will need even more help making the transition from the hospital to home. And the JCAHO will look more closely than ever at the clinical record for proof of adequate discharge planning.

### Intervention

During this phase of the nursing process, you'll carry out or delegate the interventions outlined in the care plan. Start this phase as soon as the patient has a documented care plan, working with him and his family to perform the designated interventions and move toward the desired outcomes. Document your interventions in your progress notes. You can supplement these notes with flow sheets.

### Evaluation

During this phase, you'll determine whether the desired outcomes have been reached. To do so, review the clinical record. For example, you may examine a care plan that calls for a patient to lose 2 lb a week. The progress notes show that he was taught about dietary modifications and that he was weighed a week later. The assessment flow sheet shows a 2-lb weight loss. Thus, you know that the desired outcome was achieved. If you found that the patient lost only 1 lb, you'd have to determine why and modify the care plan accordingly.

Once you've evaluated the outcome, you'll need to document it in your progress notes with clear evaluative statements that demonstrate the patient's progress toward the desired outcomes. (See *Writing clear evaluative statements.*) This step has become increasingly important because the JCAHO, PROs, insurance companies, and others examine such progress notes carefully, looking for positive patient outcomes and the measures taken to prevent complications.

CHECKLIST

### Writing clear evaluative statements

Below you'll find examples of clear evaluative statements describing common outcomes. Notice how each one uses specific details, not general statements.

☐ *Response to p.r.n. medication*
"States relief of pain 10 minutes after receiving I.V. morphine."
"Wheezing and shortness of breath subsided 5 minutes after receiving inhalation of albuterol."

☐ *Response to patient teaching*
"Able to describe the signs and symptoms of hyperglycemia and hypoglycemia."
"Despite three attempts, patient couldn't adequately demonstrate self-injection of insulin."

☐ *Tolerance of changes or increases in activity*
"Able to walk 15 feet on crutches with correct technique."

☐ *Ability to perform activities of daily living, particularly those that influence discharge planning*
"Unable to feed self independently because of muscle tremor."
"Requires a walker to get to bathroom."

☐ *Tolerance of treatments*
"Tolerated dressing change with no complaint of pain."
"Skin became pink and respirations grew less labored (16/minute) after receiving 4 liters/minute of nasal oxygen for 10 minutes."

## Nursing documentation formats

All your patient care documentation should follow the nursing process, but the format you use will vary with the health care facility where you work. Some facilities still use traditional narrative charting; others have switched to problem-oriented charting or even newer formats, such as Focus charting, PIE charting, and charting by exception. (See *Comparing documentation formats,* pages 16 and 17.)

### Narrative charting
Primarily used with the source-oriented clinical record, narrative charting consists of a straightforward, chronologic account of the patient's status, nursing interventions performed, and the patient's response to those interventions. It's usually recorded on the progress notes. Flow sheets commonly supplement these narrative notes.

Although such charting is simple, it takes a great deal of time. It also results in an unstructured record, making it difficult to quickly determine the patient's progress.

### Problem-oriented charting
Stemming from the POMR system, this type of charting focuses on the patient's problems and provides a structure that's absent from narrative charting. As mentioned earlier, progress notes are organized according to the SOAP framework:
• Subjective data: information the patient tells you
• Objective data: information you gather by observation
• Assessment: your conclusions about the patient's problem, based on the subjective and objective data
• Plan: the proposed interventions to resolve the problem.

SOAPIE notes, a modification of SOAP notes, include two more components:
• Intervention: the interventions you perform to resolve the problem
• Evaluation: your evaluation of the patient's response to interventions.

You can also use flow sheets to supplement this approach. As with the POMR approach, problem-oriented charting has the drawback of requiring elaborate notations even for simple patient problems.

### Focus charting
With this approach, information is organized by key words listed in one column. These key words may be a sign or symptom (such as pain), a nursing diagnosis (such as potential for infection), a behavior, a condition, a significant event, or an acute change in the patient's condition. In the next column, you organize your notes according to the DAR framework: record the corresponding *data* you gather while observing the patient, the *actions* you take, and the patient's *response.*

Although complex, this system requires fewer notations than the SOAPIE system. Some nurses also believe this system makes it easier to document the nursing process in general and nursing diagnoses in particular.

### PIE charting
As originally designed, PIE charting consisted of a running list of nursing diagnoses, each with a progress note. Each entry was divided into three components: the problem, labeled P, written as a nursing diagnosis; the interventions, labeled I, stating the nursing actions taken to alleviate the problem; and the evaluation, labeled E, a determination of the success of the nursing interventions. A variation of this format, APIE notes include a fourth component for assessment findings, listed before the problem component and labeled A.

A logical, easy-to-use format, APIE charting permits you to document according to the nursing process. But it doesn't provide a central point for documenting planned care. To find all the nursing actions performed for each problem, you'd have to read several shifts' worth of documentation—a major drawback to APIE charting.

## Charting by exception

With this method, you document only significant findings or exceptions to certain norms. These norms are based on clearly defined standards of practice and predetermined criteria for nursing assessments and interventions. You document explanations of exceptions to the norm in longhand notes on the progress notes. Specially designed flow sheets used for documenting physical assessments and interventions supplement these notes.

Although more involved than the Focus approach, charting by exception still streamlines documentation and saves time.

## Computerized documentation

Along with the evolution of new formats comes another development: the change from the handwritten to the computerized clinical record. If you haven't switched to computerized nursing documentation already, you may in the near future.

Of course, health care facilities have used computers for payroll, billing, patient bed assignments, pharmacy orders, and other auxiliary needs for years. Many facilities use specially designed software programs called hospital information systems (HISs) to link various departments electronically. But

nursing departments are typically among the last to use computers to meet their needs.

Why? Largely because software programs that can handle the complex requirements of nursing departments have only recently become available. Also, until recently, nurses couldn't agree on the type of information to include in such programs. And, despite their size, nursing departments usually haven't wielded much power within health care facilities.

But now, progressive health care facilities document patient care with computerized nursing information systems (NISs). These systems let you perform such varied tasks as generating Kardex forms, nursing work sheets, vital sign reports, and nursing care plans; charting assessment data, progress notes, medication administration, and intake and output; and writing and storing nursing management reports.

### Benefits of computers

Computers not only store a large amount of information and allow quick access to it, they also can help provide confidentiality and speed up the documentation process.

*Information storage.* A large mainframe computer can store an enormous amount of data—enough for all the departments in a health care facility. Personal computers or terminals located at work stations throughout a facility allow access to that information. Recently, several U.S. hospitals have added terminals right at patients' bedsides, making access even easier. (See *Using bedside computer terminals,* page 18.)

*Confidentiality.* To gain access to a patient's computerized clinical rec-

*(Text continues on page 18.)*

## Comparing documentation formats

Below you'll find examples of four documentation formats, each showing the same nursing actions—administering an analgesic to a patient with abdominal pain and assessing his reaction to the medication.

You won't find an example of charting by exception—a fifth charting format—because the patient responded as he should have to the pain medication and, as the format's name implies, you only chart exceptions to the expected response. If you were using charting by exception, you'd record the analgesic administration on the medication administration record.

### Narrative charting

| Date | Time | Progress notes |
|------|------|----------------|
| 1/20/92 | 10:00 a.m. | Grimacing and complaining of burning in abdomen; Demerol 75 mg I.M. administered——— Mary Norris, RN |
| | 10:45 a.m. | Expressed relief of pain——— Mary Norris, RN |

### Problem-oriented (SOAPIE) charting

| Date | Time | Progress notes |
|------|------|----------------|
| 1/20/92 | 10:00 a.m. | S: "My stomach is burning." O: Grimacing, rubbing abdomen A: Abdominal pain P: Administer analgesic I: Demerol 75 mg I.M. Mary Norris, RN |
| | 10:45 a.m. | E: Expressed relief of pain——— Mary Norris, RN |

**Focus charting**

| Date | Time | Focus | Patient care notes |
|------|------|-------|--------------------|
| 1/20/92 | 10:00 a.m. | Pain | D: Grimacing, complains of burning in abdomen |
| | | | A: Demerol 75 mg I.M.———— Mary Norris, RN |
| | 10:45 a.m. | | R: Expressed relief of pain ———— Mary Norris, RN |

**PIE charting**

| Date | Time | Remarks |
|------|------|---------|
| 1/20/92 | 10:00 a.m. | A#1 Expressed abdominal pain. |
| | | P #1 Pain related to abdominal surgery. |
| | 10:45 a.m. | I#1 Demerol 75 mg I.M. Mary Norris RN |
| | | E#1 Expressed relief of pain ———— Mary Norris RN |

## Using bedside computer terminals

A bedside computer terminal lets you document as soon as you complete an action or make an observation, eliminating the need to write on a work sheet and later copy the information on the patient's chart. Such a terminal also lets you retrieve information instantly. And with one terminal at bedside and one at the nurses' station, you can, in effect, keep the chart in both places at once.

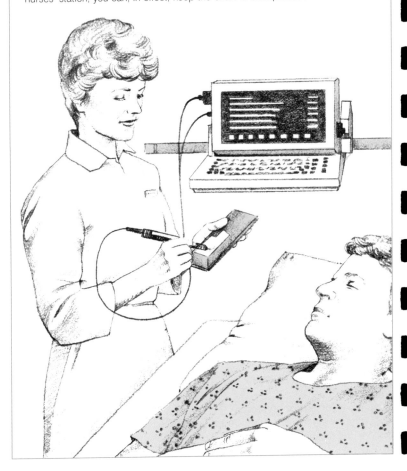

ord, a health care team member first must enter the proper identification code. These codes may even specify the type of information that a particular team member may have. For example, a dietitian may be as-signed a code that allows her to see only diet orders and the patient's nutrition history, but not physical therapy information. Although these codes can help maintain a patient's right to privacy, if they're misused, his right can still be violated.

*Rapid documentation.* To use a computer system for documentation, you'll simply enter a code or the patient's name to bring the patient's chart onto the screen. Then you can choose the function you want to perform. For example, you can enter new data on the nursing care plan or progress notes, or pull up all vital signs for comparison — all more quickly than you could with traditional documentation.

Depending on which type of computer your health care facility has and what kind of software it runs, the computer may allow you to enter information using a keyboard, a light pen, a touch-sensitive screen, a mouse, or even your voice. Most computerized care plan systems provide you with a selection of words or phrases you can choose from to individualize documentation on standardized formats. In some systems, you can use a series of phrases to quickly create a complete narrative note. You can then elaborate on a problem or clarify flow sheet documentation in the comment section of a computerized form by entering standardized phrases or typing in comments.

Computers have several other advantages — and disadvantages, too. (See *Using the computer: Pros and cons,* page 20.)

## Nursing information systems

NIS software programs allow you to record nursing actions in the electronic record, making nursing documentation easier. These systems reflect most or all of the components of the nursing process so they can meet the standards of the ANA and the JCAHO. What's more, each NIS provides different features and can be customized to conform to a facili-

ty's documentation forms and formats.

Currently, most NISs manage information passively. They can collect, transmit, organize, format, and print data and can display information you can use to make a decision. But most NISs don't suggest decisions for you. Some of the newer systems, however, can suggest nursing diagnoses based on predefined assessment data that you enter. The more sophisticated systems provide you with standardized patient status and nursing intervention phrases that you can use to construct your progress notes. These systems let you change these standardized phrases, if necessary, and allow room for you to add your own notes.

*New developments.* The most recent NISs interact with you, prompting you with questions and suggestions about the information you enter. Ultimately, this computerized sequential decision-making format can lead to more effective nursing care and documentation. Such a system requires you to enter only a brief narrative. The sequential questioning and diagnostic suggestions the system provides make your documentation thorough — and quick. Yet, the program allows you to add or change information as needed, making your documentation fit your patient.

## Nursing minimum data set

Still under development, the nursing minimum data set (NMDS) will attempt to standardize nursing information. It will contain information on nursing care, patient demographics, and hospitals (such as lengths of hospitalizations). Because the NMDS will contain information on nursing care nationwide, it will allow a com-

## Using the computer: Pros and cons

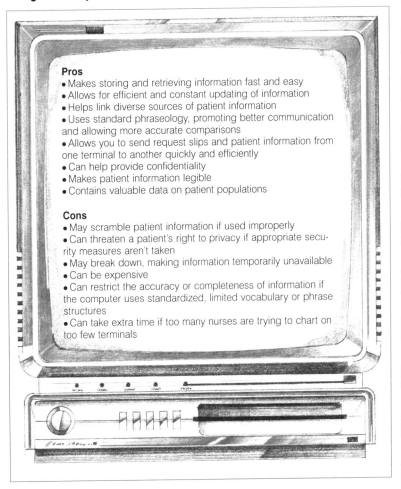

**Pros**
- Makes storing and retrieving information fast and easy
- Allows for efficient and constant updating of information
- Helps link diverse sources of patient information
- Uses standard phraseology, promoting better communication and allowing more accurate comparisons
- Allows you to send request slips and patient information from one terminal to another quickly and efficiently
- Can help provide confidentiality
- Makes patient information legible
- Contains valuable data on patient populations

**Cons**
- May scramble patient information if used improperly
- Can threaten a patient's right to privacy if appropriate security measures aren't taken
- May break down, making information temporarily unavailable
- Can be expensive
- Can restrict the accuracy or completeness of information if the computer uses standardized, limited vocabulary or phrase structures
- Can take extra time if too many nurses are trying to chart on too few terminals

parison of nursing data from different clinical settings, patient populations, and geographic areas. And because it will contain information about patient care over time, it can demonstrate trends in nursing care.

But the NMDS will do more than provide valuable information for research and policy making. It will also help you provide better patient care. For instance, examining the outcomes of patient populations will help you set realistic outcomes for your patient. Plus, the NMDS can help you formulate accurate nursing diagnoses and plan interventions.

The standardized format of the NMDS will also lead to more consistent nursing documentation. With this system, all data will be coded, making documentation and information retrieval faster and easier. Currently, NANDA is including numerical codes on all nursing diagnoses so they can be used with the NMDS.

### Related computer functions
Computers can also help you complete nurse management reports, provide patient classification data, and make staffing projections. They can identify patient education needs and supply data for nursing research and education. And some bedside terminals can measure vital signs electronically.

# Current challenges in nursing documentation

Today, documenting accurately has become more important than ever. As discussed, clinical records must stand up to close scrutiny by quality assurance committees, insurance companies, and lawyers as well as professional standards and accrediting committees. Also, the sheer number of health care professionals who may care for a single patient increases the need for accurate documentation. One patient may need the services of a laboratory technician, a physical therapist, a respiratory therapist, a dietitian, a pharmacist, a private doctor, and several consultants, interns, and residents. Plus, the patient may need nursing care not only from the nurses on the unit, but also from flex-time and agency nurses, nurse specialists, discharge planners, nurse supervisors, and case managers. All these team members must know what

## Documenting accurately

To ensure accuracy, ask yourself these questions as you document:
☐ *Have I recorded the exact time?* If the patient complains of pain at 12:05 a.m., write "12:05 a.m."—not "approximately 12:00." Noting the precise times of a significant complaint and of your response may prove crucial, especially in a court of law.
☐ *Have I documented the exact distance?* Don't chart that a patient with a cerebrovascular accident "can walk to the door and back." That won't mean anything to a nurse unfamiliar with the patient's room—a home health nurse, for example. She needs to know the actual distance the patient can walk so she can plan safe home care.
☐ *Have I documented the exact amount?* For example, when caring for a patient with a fluid and electrolyte imbalance, measure and record the exact amount of vomitus. Don't use subjective terms, such as "a small amount." The precise measurement may be critical.
☐ *Have I given a precise description?* Don't write "incision appears to be healing" after inspecting a patient's surgical wound. Instead, use specific details. For instance, you might say, "Wound on left dorsal foot measures 7 cm × 2 cm. Pink granulation tissue at wound edges; no drainage noted."

care the patient is receiving from the other team members. So your documentation must communicate clearly. (See *Documenting accurately*.)

You not only have to document clearly, you also have to document quickly. Current constraints on reimbursement are forcing administrators to investigate all possible cost containment measures, includ-

## Meeting documentation goals

When you document, you want to record information accurately and save time. The chart below gives you an overview of which measures can help you accomplish these two goals.

| MEASURE | PROMOTES ACCURACY | SAVES TIME |
|---|---|---|
| Follow the nursing process. | ✓ | |
| Use nursing diagnoses. | ✓ | |
| Use flow sheets. | ✓ | ✓ |
| Document at bedside. | ✓ | ✓ |
| Individualize your charting. | ✓ | |
| Don't repeat information. | | ✓ |
| Sign off with initials. | | ✓ |
| Don't document for other caregivers. | ✓ | ✓ |
| Use computerized documentation. | ✓ | ✓ |
| Use fax machines. | ✓ | ✓ |

ing improving nursing productivity. Other factors — the nursing shortage, sicker patients, the demands of using complex equipment, and the expanding role of nurses — put more pressure on you to manage your time as efficiently as possible. All this calls for you to document more rapidly.

### Meeting the challenges

How can you document more accurately and quickly? The following suggestions will help. (See *Meeting documentation goals.*)

*Follow the nursing process.* As explained, this problem-solving process provides the framework for quality care. Your documentation can best substantiate quality care if it reflects this process. And the re-

sulting logical, complete, and well-organized record will help other caregivers provide quality care.

*Use nursing diagnoses.* Using standardized diagnostic labels to identify actual or potential health problems will result in less confusion and better care. Depending on your health care facility's policy, you may be required to use nursing diagnoses.

*Document frequently and immediately.* If you chart during your shift — right after you make an observation or intervene — rather than at the end of your shift, you'll document more accurately and forget less information. You'll also provide other team members with the most current information on the patient's care and progress. Flow sheets help you keep your documentation current, as does bedside charting. A growing number of health care facilities are requiring immediate documentation.

**Individualize your charting.** Documenting the same information for all patients with the same diagnosis neither promotes accuracy nor demonstrates quality care. Make sure your charting demonstrates the particular care that each patient received.

**Don't repeat information.** Not only does this waste time, but it can be misleading. If you record data on a flow sheet, don't repeat it in the progress notes. Instead, use the progress notes to clarify information on the flow sheet or to add data, such as psychosocial information or follow-up care, that you can't chart on a flow sheet.

**Sign off with initials.** If the policy at your facility allows, you can save time by signing your name, licensure, and initials on a flow sheet near the front of the chart, then using only your initials thereafter.

**Don't document for other caregivers.** Doctors should regularly document their own progress notes, as should physical and respiratory therapists and other health care team members. Don't feel responsible for recording routine doctor visits or care provided by other team members.

**Use the Kardex effectively.** Used informally for decades, the patient care Kardex (sometimes called the nursing record) gives you a quick presentation of basic patient care information. You'll typically refer to the Kardex during change-of-shift

reports and several times throughout the day to quickly review patient information. Kardexes come in various shapes and sizes and may even be generated by a computer. (See *Components of a Kardex cover sheet,* pages 24 and 25.) You'll find the following information on a typical Kardex:

• patient's name, age, and religion
• medical diagnoses, listed by priority
• current medical orders for medication and treatments, diet, I.V. therapy, and tests
• permitted activities, functional limitations, assistance needed, and safety precautions.

A Kardex can be made more effective by tailoring the information to the needs of a particular setting. For instance, a home care Kardex should have information on family contacts, doctors, other services, and emergency referrals.

If the Kardex is included in the clinical record at your facility, you can save charting time because you won't need to repeat the information in another part of the record. Make sure you write in ink, revising information when the doctor writes new orders or the patient's needs change. In some facilities, the Kardex has been eliminated, and its information has been incorporated into the nursing care plan.

**Use computerized documentation.** You've already seen how computers can help you document more efficiently and quickly. Although not widespread yet, computer documentation will become more common as costs decrease, equipment becomes easier to use, and better programs are developed.

**Use fax machines.** These machines
*(Text continues on page 26.)*

## Components of a Kardex cover sheet

Below you'll find the kind of information that might be included on the cover sheet of a patient care Kardex for a medical-surgical unit. Inside the Kardex, which is folded in half horizontally, you'll find further patient care information.

**Care status**
Self-care ☐
Partial care with assist ☐
Complete care ☐
Shower ☐
Tub ☐
Active exercises ☐
Passive exercises ☐

**Special**
Back care ☐
Mouth care ☐
Foot care ☐
Perineal care ☐
Catheter care ☐
Trach care ☐
Other:

**Condition**
Satisfactory ☐
Fair ☐
Guarded ☐
Critical ☐
No code ☐
Date:

**Prosthesis**
Dentures ☐
Contact lenses ☐
Eye ☐
Other:

**Isolation**
Strict ☐
Wound and skin ☐
Respiratory ☐
Hepatitis ☐
Enteric ☐
Other:

**Diet**
Type:
Force fluids ☐
NPO ☐
Assist with feeding ☐
Isolation tray ☐

**Admission**
Height:
Weight:
BP:
TPR:

**Frequency**
BP:
TPR:
Apical pulse:
Weight:
Neuro check:
Monitor:
Strips:
Turn:
Cough:
Deep breathe:
Central venous
   pressure:
Other:

**GI tubes**
Salem sump ☐
Levin tube ☐
Other:

**Respiratory therapy**
Oxygen ☐
Liters/minute:
Method:
  Nebulizer ☐
  Chest PT ☐
  Incentive spirometry ☐
  Ventilator ☐
  T-piece ☐
Other:

**Feedings**

**Activity**
Bed rest ☐
Chair ☐
Chair with restraint ☐
Dangle ☐
Commode ☐
Commode assist ☐
Ambulate ☐
BRP ☐
Other:

**Mode of transport**
Wheelchair ☐
Stretcher ☐

**I.V. devices**
Heparin lock ☐
Peripheral I.V. ☐
Subclavian I.V. ☐
Total or partial parenteral ☐
nutrition

**Irrigations**

**Dressings**
Type:
Change:

| **Drains**<br>Type:<br>Number: | **Restraints**<br>Type:<br>Constant ☐<br>PRN ☐<br>Nights ☐ | **Stools** |
| **Urine output**<br>I & O ☐<br>Strain urine ☐<br>Indwelling catheter ☐<br>Continuous bladder ☐<br>  irrigation | **24-hour collection** | **Special notes** |
| **Side rails**<br>Constant ☐<br>PRN ☐<br>Nights ☐ | | **Social services** |

The format and specific information on a Kardex will vary with the needs of the patient population. For instance, the cover sheet of a patient care Kardex on a critical care unit would include the same basic information already shown plus information specific to the unit, including the following:

| **Monitoring**<br>Hardwire ☐<br>Telemetry ☐<br>Pulmonary artery line ☐<br>  Pulmonary artery<br>  pressure: | Pulmonary capillary wedge<br>  pressure:<br><br>Arterial line ☐<br>Other: | **Mechanical ventilation**<br>Tidal volume:<br>$FIO_2$:<br>Mode:<br>Rate: |

On an obstetrics unit, you might find the following additional information on the Kardex cover sheet:

| **Delivery**<br>Date:<br>Time:<br>Type of delivery:<br><br>**Special procedures**<br>Peri-lite ☐<br>Sitz bath ☐<br>Witch hazel compress ☐<br>Breast binders ☐<br>Ice ☐<br>Abdominal binders ☐<br>Other: | **Mother**<br>Due date:<br>Gravida:<br>Para:<br>Rh:<br>Blood type:<br>Membranes ruptured:<br>Episiotomy ☐<br>Lacerations ☐<br>RhoGAM ☐<br>  studies<br>Rubella titer ☐ | **Infant**<br>Male ☐<br>Female ☐<br>Full term ☐<br>Premature ☐<br>Nursing ☐<br>Formula ☐<br>Condition:<br><br><br>Other: |

can improve communication dramatically. Fax machines on nursing units and in other hospital departments allow you to send and receive orders, documentation forms, patient records, and test results quickly. And machines in doctors' offices can save you from taking and documenting orders over the phone.

---

## Suggested readings

*Accreditation Manual for Hospitals.* Chicago: Joint Commission on Accreditation of Healthcare Organizations, 1991.

Atkinson, L.D., and Murray, M.E. *Understanding the Nursing Process: Fundamentals of Care Planning,* 4th ed. New York: Pergamon Press, 1990.

Courtright, G. "Unofficial Charting: Make It Work for You," *Nursing Management* 19(1):62, January 1988.

Hines, G.L. "DRGs: Nursing Documentation Contributes to the Bottom Line," *Nursing Clinics of North America* 23(3):579-86, September 1988.

Morton, P.G. *Health Assessment in Nursing.* Springhouse, Pa.: Springhouse Corp., 1989.

Werley, H., and Lang, N. *Identification of the Nursing Minimum Data Set.* New York: Springer Publishing Co., 1988.

# 2
# LEGAL ASPECTS OF DOCUMENTATION

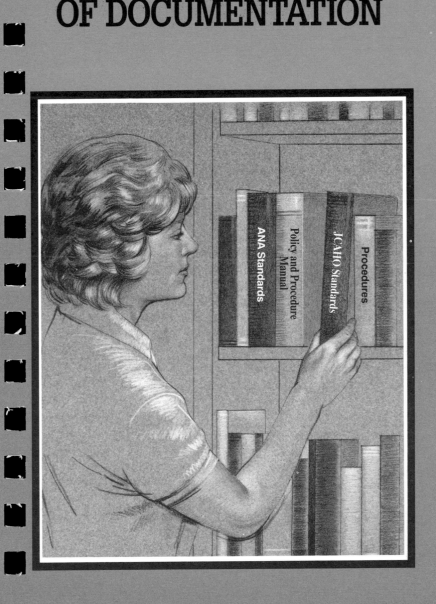

ANA Standards

Policy and Procedure Manual

JCAHO Standards

Procedures

An important legal document, the clinical record can provide useful information for patient competency hearings, personal injury lawsuits, and work-related disability claims. Of course, the clinical record also serves as a key element in litigation for medical malpractice and negligence claims.

Because your progress notes and flow sheets describe patient activities, the courts commonly focus on these portions of the clinical record to support or dispute claims. So your documentation needs to be complete and accurate.

To ensure that it is, first review the laws and regulations, professional standards, and policies and procedures governing documentation. Then review the guidelines for documenting in accordance with these rules.

# Rules governing documentation

To protect yourself legally, you need to follow the established rules of documentation. These rules come from federal regulations, state and provincial statutes, standards set by professional organizations and accreditation boards, policies and procedures of your health care facility, and case law precedents.

### Federal regulations
You need to document your care based on federal regulations from several agencies. These regulations cover issues ranging from workers' compensation to quality assurance. The Health Care Financing Administration (HCFA), for instance, requires documentation of mortality rates related to specific procedures a patient undergoes. This information then allows an analysis of the quality of patient care.

Other federal regulations set standards for participation in Medicare and Medicaid. These regulations stipulate the form and content of the clinical record. Medicare regulations mandate that adequate clinical records be kept for all patients and that these records contain specific information to justify the diagnosis and treatment provided. Although regulations for Medicare don't have the authority of law, most health care facilities follow them to ensure their eligibility for federal funds.

Periodically, Medicare administrators update the requirements for program participation—called *conditions of participation*. Health care facilities respond to the conditions of participation by completing new HCFA administration forms.

### State and provincial laws
Although specific regulations vary, all states and Canadian provinces require health care facilities to keep records documenting patient care. Some states set forth specific guidelines in their nurse practice acts. In Canada, each province provides guidelines in its public hospital act.

Basically, states require documentation of births, deaths, and infectious diseases. The development of specific guidelines and requirements falls primarily to professional organizations such as the American Nurses' Association (ANA) and the Joint Commission on Accreditation of Healthcare Organizations (JCAHO).

### Professional standards
ANA and JCAHO standards are much more stringent than any state law.

***ANA standards.*** The ANA's Standards of Nursing Practice stipulate that documentation should be based on the nursing process, that it should be continuous, and that it should be accessible to all members of the health care team.

When developing practice standards, the ANA polls its national membership. Because the standards represent a national consensus, they carry a great deal of authority in court. Thus, in a legal dispute, your record of your actions will be compared to the expected level of practice, as defined by the national standards. If your documentation doesn't show that your actions met these standards, you may be liable.

***JCAHO standards.*** A key authority in accrediting health care facilities, JCAHO sets widely accepted professional practice and documentation standards. The practice standards can be used to judge how well a specific patient need was met. And documenting according to JCAHO standards helps ensure your facility's accreditation.

JCAHO standards don't mandate a particular format for documentation. But JCAHO does require each health care facility to adopt a standard format that conforms to JCAHO standards. When you correctly use forms based on JCAHO standards, you can be sure you've met the accepted standard of practice for documentation. For example, to meet JCAHO standards for discharge planning, you must address the patient's continuing care and referrals made for that care. Although JCAHO has no specific form to demonstrate conformity with this standard, a health care facility's form that meets JCAHO standards will address these points. The form will also remind you to address all aspects of discharge planning.

JCAHO also requires you to document a patient's ability to care for himself, such as his ability to perform activities of daily living. (See *Documenting self-care capabilities,* page 30.) You must also document a patient's readiness for discharge under JCAHO standards. From a legal perspective, the importance of documenting this information can't be overstated. Under the diagnosis-related groups (DRGs) system, patients can easily be discharged prematurely and possibly injured as a result. Thus, thorough documentation of a patient's readiness for discharge and his ability to perform postdischarge activities are more important now than ever. Your documentation can either support or refute a patient's claim that his injury resulted from a premature discharge or a lack of proper discharge instructions.

## Policies and procedures

In all likelihood, your facility has integrated the pertinent regulations, laws, and standards covering documentation into its own policy and procedure manual, giving you a set of standardized guidelines. The manual should identify the staff members responsible for documenting each part of a patient's clinical record, as well as the charting techniques and procedures that meet the appropriate standard of care.

Be sure you know and carefully follow your facility's policies and procedures. In a trial, the patient's lawyer will use documentation to try to prove that the standard of care wasn't met. A complete clinical record gives you hard evidence that it was met.

## Applying standards of care

The case of *Pisel v. Stamford Com-*

## Documenting self-care capabilities

Forms for documenting a patient's ability to care for himself vary among facilities. But all forms have one common goal: to ensure that your documentation meets the requirements of the JCAHO.

This sample form indicates that the patient can bathe, dress, eat, and turn by himself, though he needs help transferring from one position to another and walking. The patient also uses a walker and has upper and lower dentures, eyeglasses, and a hearing aid.

### ACTIVITIES OF DAILY LIVING

| Activities | Independent | With assistance | Totally dependent |
|---|---|---|---|
| Bathing | ✔ | | |
| Dressing | ✔ | | |
| Eating | ✔ | | |
| Transferring | | ✔ | |
| Turning | ✔ | | |
| Walking | | ✔ | |

**ASSISTIVE DEVICES:** Cane _____ Walker __✔__ Crutches _____
    Splint: R _____ L _____ Brace: R _____ L _____
**DENTURE:** Upper __✔__ Lower __✔__
**CONTACT LENS:** R _____ L _____
**EYEGLASSES** __✔__
**HEARING AID** __✔__
**PROSTHESIS:** Arm: R _____ L _____ Leg: R _____ L _____
    Eye: R _____ L _____ Other _____

*munity Hospital* shows how courts consider local, state, and national standards of care. In this case, nurses at a mental health hospital left a young, psychotic patient unattended in a locked seclusion room. The patient forcibly wedged her head between the bed frame and side rail and suffered permanent neurologic damage. The patient's relatives sued the nurses and the hospital for malpractice. In the absence of hospital policies that might have applied in this case, the court relied on the testimony of an expert witness as well as on ANA standards and federal regulations to judge the nurses' care.

The court found the nurses and the hospital guilty of violating applicable standards of care, based on the following:

• failure to remove a steel bed from a seclusion room
• failure to constantly observe the patient
• failure to completely assess the patient's status
• failure to notify the attending psychiatrist of the patient's acutely psychotic condition
• failure to implement medical orders.

Further evidence revealed that someone had destroyed the nurses' notes describing the incident and then created new ones. The falsified record proved that those responsible were conscious of their negligence.

# Guidelines for documentation

You can help avoid legal problems by following certain general guidelines for documentation. For example, you should document accurately, completely, and objectively. Also, you should be sure to fill out each documentation form properly.

## Document accurately

Record the facts — not opinions or assumptions. Never falsify the clinical record to cover up a negligent act. A false record discovered during litigation can destroy the credibility of the entire clinical record. Not only could this influence the verdict, but a falsification could result in the award of punitive damages — which may not be covered by your malpractice insurance.

## Document completely

Although you don't need to chart routine tasks, such as changing bed linens, you do need to chart all relevant information relating to patient care and reflecting the nursing process. In court, you'll find it difficult to prove that you provided an aspect of patient care if you haven't documented it. For the best legal protection, completely document actual or potential problems, nursing actions taken to resolve or prevent them, and the patient's response to your actions. (For more information, see *When in doubt, chart everything,* page 32.)

The case of *Villetto v. Weilbaecher* illustrates the need for complete documentation. In this case, the nurses noticed that the patient had developed several blisters while recovering from surgery for a fractured kneecap. Each nurse recorded her observations in the nurses' progress notes and reported the blisters to the doctor. The patient later sued the doctor for failing to treat the blisters. The doctor couldn't defend himself successfully because his record (the doctor's progress notes) didn't mention blisters until 6 days after the nurses documented them.

## Note the time

Be specific about times in the chart. In particular, note the exact time of all sudden changes, significant events, and nursing actions. Avoid block charting such as "7 a.m. to 3 p.m." This sounds vague and implies inattention to the patient. For these reasons, block charting has been prohibited by some state health departments.

Also try to document pertinent information as soon as possible after an event. That way, you won't be as likely to forget important details, and your charting will be more accurate and clinically useful. Plus, if you become involved in litigation, you'll find it easier to defend your

## When in doubt, chart everything

As you know, you need to chart your nursing observations and interventions. But you may not be sure what other information you should record.

To be on the safe side, you should chart as much factual information about your patient's care as possible. In particular, you should note:
• incidents
• omitted treatments
• implementation of safety precautions
• attempts to reach the doctor.

### Case in point
Failing to record any of this information invites misunderstandings and jeopardizes the quality of the patient's care. Consider this example.

The doctor's orders for Mrs. Cauthen state: "Out of bed for 20 minutes, three times daily, as tolerated."

After explaining the doctor's plan to Mrs. Cauthen, a nurse helps her out of bed. But, as soon as the nurse helps her to her feet, Mrs. Cauthen drops to her knees. She's not hurt but appears angry. She says she fell because the nurse made her get out of bed. The nurse gets Mrs. Cauthen back in bed, assesses her for injuries, and hears her say she's not hurt. Then, without charting the incident, notifying the doctor, or completing an incident report, the nurse leaves to care for another patient.

Two hours later, a different nurse reads Mrs. Cauthen's chart and assumes she hasn't been out of bed. Again, as soon as Mrs. Cauthen tries to stand, she collapses. But this time, she fractures her hip.

Mrs. Cauthen complains to the doctor about her two falls, and the doctor immediately notifies the nursing supervisor about the undocumented incident. The hospital places the first nurse on probation for something she considered a minor charting omission. However, had Mrs. Cauthen sued the hospital, the nurse would have been facing a malpractice charge.

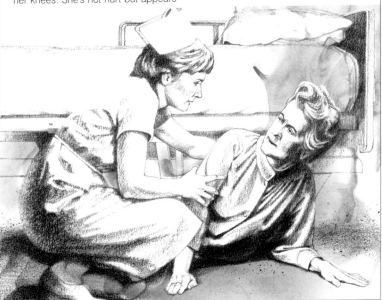

actions because prompt charting leaves no question as to when an event occurred. If you can't document at once, note the time when you do chart, explain the delay (for example, "chart not available"), and note the time the event occurred.

## Document objectively

Record exactly what you see, hear, and do. When you record a patient's statement, use his exact words.

Avoid making subjective statements such as: "Patient's level of cooperation has deteriorated since yesterday." Instead, include the facts that led you to this conclusion. For example, write: "The patient stated, 'I don't want to learn how to inject insulin. I tried yesterday, but I'm not going to do it today.'" (See *Comparing subjective and objective charting,* page 34.) In some cases, you may include your conclusion, as long as you record the objective assessment data that supports it.

Remember to document only data you witness yourself, or data from a reliable source—such as the patient or another nurse. When you include information reported by someone else, cite your source.

## Avoid assigning blame

Never use the clinical record to vent anger or assign blame. Avoid judgmental statements such as: "The patient failed to receive his therapy because staff was at lunch."

Also avoid recording unnecessary or unrelated information—such as statements about staffing shortages—that could be misconstrued in court as having a bearing on a patient's condition. Such a shortage, for instance, may or may not have had a direct effect on a patient.

## Fill out the form correctly

When you document your care,

make sure you use the appropriate form, fill it out in ink, sign each entry, use standard abbreviations, spell correctly, and write legibly. Also correct errors properly, write on every line of the form, note omissions on the form, co-sign it correctly, and identify the patient on every page of the form.

***Use appropriate forms.*** Be sure to use the forms required by your facility's policy and procedure manual. If, for instance, the manual directs you to use a neurologic flow sheet, you should use it instead of describing a patient's neurologic status in your progress notes. Such a flow sheet helps you document accurately and reminds you to cover all the elements of a complete neurologic assessment.

A jury faced with a properly completed flow sheet will have little doubt that you performed a complete neurologic assessment. But failure to use an approved form may raise questions as to whether you followed your facility's policy and met the standards of care.

***Write in ink.*** Because it's a permanent document, the clinical record should be completed in ink or printed out from a computer. Use only black or blue ink, if possible; green and red ink (the colors traditionally used on evening and night shifts) don't photocopy well. Also don't use felt-tipped pens on forms with carbons; the pens may not produce sufficient pressure for copies.

***Sign each entry.*** Be sure to sign each entry you make in your progress notes with your first name or initial, full last name, and professional licensure (such as RN or LPN). If you find the last entry un-

*(Text continues on page 37.)*

## Comparing subjective and objective charting

The most common charting error is using value judgments and opinions (subjective data) rather than factual information (objective data). Considered inappropriate, subjective documentation conveys what you think about the patient's condition—not information about the condition itself. Compare the following subjective entries with their objective counterparts.

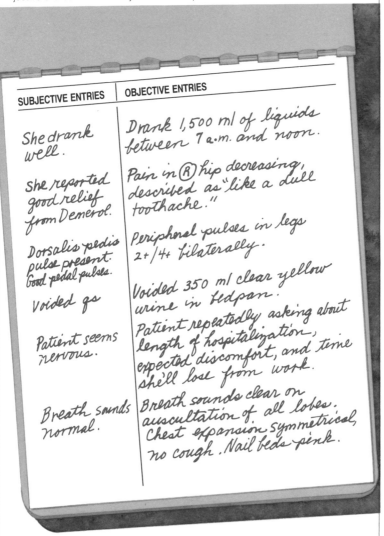

| SUBJECTIVE ENTRIES | OBJECTIVE ENTRIES |
|---|---|
| She drank well. | Drank 1,500 ml of liquids between 7 a.m. and noon. |
| She reported good relief from Demerol. | Pain in ® hip decreasing, described as "like a dull toothache." |
| Dorsalis pedis pulse present. Good pedal pulses. | Peripheral pulses in legs 2+/4+ bilaterally. |
| Voided qs | Voided 350 ml clear yellow urine in bedpan. |
| Patient seems nervous. | Patient repeatedly asking about length of hospitalization, expected discomfort, and time she'll lose from work. |
| Breath sounds normal. | Breath sounds clear on auscultation of all lobes. Chest expansion symmetrical, no cough. Nail beds pink. |

CHARTING

## Signing nurses' notes

To discourage others from adding information to the nurses' notes, draw a line through any blank spaces and sign your name to the far right of the column.

> P: Will continue plan and request diabetic nurse special-ist to assess patient's knowledge of diabetes mellitus on the 3rd or 4th postop day.————J. Rice, RN

If you don't have enough room to sign your name after the last word of your entry, draw a line from the last word to the end of the line. Then, drop down to the next line and draw a line from the left margin toward the right margin, leaving room to sign your name on the far right side.

> and hypoglycemia. A: Excellent know-ledge of disease and management. P: See no need for additional follow up.————J. Rice RN

If you want to record a lot of information but think you'll run out of room on the page, leave space at the bottom of the page to write "Continued on next page" and add your signature. Start the next page with "Continued from previous page." Then finish your notes and sign the second page as usual.

> return demonstration. medication effective. Patient drowsy and (continued on next page)————J. Rice RN

PROGRESS NOTES

> (continued from pre-vious page) relaxed on departure for OR. ————J. Rice, RN

## Abbreviations to avoid

The JCAHO requires every health care facility to develop a list of approved abbreviations for staff use. But certain abbreviations should *never* be used because they're easily misunderstood, especially when handwritten. Here's a list of abbreviations to avoid.

| ABBREVIATION | MISINTERPRETATION | CORRECTION |
|---|---|---|
| **Apothecaries' symbols**<br><br>ʒ<br>fluidounce<br><br>ʒ<br>fluidram<br><br>ɱ<br>minim<br><br>ʒ<br>scruple | Frequently misinterpreted | Use the metric equivalents. |
| a U<br>*auris uterque*<br>each ear | Frequently misinterpreted as "OU" (*oculus uterque* – each eye) | Write it out. |
| **Drug names**<br>MTX<br>methotrexate | mustargen (mechlorethamine hydrochloride) | Use the complete spelling for drug names. |
| CPZ<br>Compazine (prochlorperazine) | chlorpromazine | |
| HCl<br>hydrochloric acid | potassium chloride ("H" is misinterpreted as "K") | |
| DIG<br>digoxin | digitoxin | |
| MVI<br>multivitamins *without* fat-soluble vitamins | multivitamins *with* fat-soluble vitamins | |
| HCTZ<br>hydrochlorothiazide | hydrocortisone (HCT) | |
| ara-c<br>vidarabine | cytarabine (ara-C) | |
| µg<br>microgram | Frequently misinterpreted as "mg" | Use "mcg." |

## Abbreviations to avoid *(continued)*

| ABBREVIATION | MISINTERPRETATION | CORRECTION |
|---|---|---|
| *OD*<br>once daily | Frequently misinterpreted as "OD" (*oculus dexter*—right eye) | Don't abbreviate "daily." Write it out. |
| *OJ*<br>orange juice | Frequently misinterpreted as "OD" (*oculus dexter*—right eye) or "OS" (*oculus sinister*—left eye). Medications that were meant to be diluted in orange juice and given orally have been given in a patient's right or left eye. | Write it out. |
| *TID*<br>once daily | Misinterpreted as "t.i.d." | Write it out. |
| *per os*<br>orally | The "os" is frequently misinterpreted as "OS" (*oculus sinister*—left eye). | Use "P.O." or "by mouth" or "orally." |
| *q.d.*<br>every day | The period after the "q" has sometimes been misinterpreted as "i," and the drug has been given q.i.d. rather than daily. | Write it out. |
| *qn*<br>nightly or at bedtime | Misinterpreted as "qh" (every hour) | Use "hs" or "nightly." |
| *qod*<br>every other day | Misinterpreted as "q.d." (daily) or "q.i.d." | Use "q other day" or "every other day." |
| *subq*<br>subcutaneous | The "q" has been misinterpreted as every. For example, a prophylactic heparin dose meant to be given 2 hours before surgery may be given *every* 2 hours before surgery. | Use "subcut," or write out "subcutaneous." |
| *U u*<br>unit | Misinterpreted as a "0" or a "4," causing a tenfold or greater overdose. | Write it out. |

signed, immediately contact the nurse who made the entry and have her sign her name. If you can't locate her, simply write and sign your progress note. The different times and handwriting on the chart should dispel confusion as to the author. (See *Signing nurses' notes,* page 35.) On a flow sheet or medication Kardex, you can use just your initials after signing your full name and licensure in the space provided.

***Use standard abbreviations.*** JCAHO standards and many state regulations require health care facilities to use an approved abbreviations list to prevent confusion. Be sure you know and use your facility's approved abbreviations. Using unap-

CHARTING

## Correcting a charting error

When you make a mistake on the clinical record, correct it by drawing a single line through it and writing the words "mistaken entry" above or beside it. Follow these words with your initials and the date. If appropriate, briefly explain the necessity for the correction.

Be sure the mistaken entry is still readable. This indicates that you're only trying to correct a mistake, not cover it up.

| DATE | TIME | PROGRESS NOTES |
|------|------|----------------|
| 2/19/92 | 0900 | ~~Pt. walked to bathroom~~ MISTAKEN ENTRY J.R. 2/19/92 states he ~~experiences no difficulty uri-~~ J. Ross, RN ~~nating.~~ |

proved abbreviations can cause ambiguity, possibly endangering a patient's health. For example, if you use "o.d." for "once a day," another nurse may misinterpret it as "right eye," and mistakenly instill medication into the patient's eye, instead of giving it once a day. (See *Abbreviations to avoid,* pages 36 and 37.)

***Spell correctly.*** When you don't know how to spell a word, look it up in a dictionary. Misspellings on a chart can cause confusion and convey a sense of unprofessionalism to a jury scrutinizing your charts.

***Write legibly.*** Effective documentation depends on legible handwriting. Illegible writing hinders communication and can lead to errors in patient care. In litigation, illegible writing creates a poor impression, damages

credibility, and can even be interpreted as negligent care. In *Gugino v. Harvard Community Health Plan,* an expert witness complained that the progress notes were sketchy. Upon reviewing the material, the judge declared the notes totally illegible and barred their use in court.

***Correct errors.*** When you make a mistake on a chart, correct it promptly. Never erase, cover, completely scratch out, or otherwise obscure an erroneous entry because this can imply a cover-up. (See *Correcting a charting error.*)

***Write on every line.*** Don't leave blank lines on any chart; fill it in completely. If information requested doesn't apply to a particular patient, write "N/A" or draw a line through the empty space. This leaves no doubt that you addressed every part of the form and also prevents others from inserting information that could change the meaning of your original documentation.

**Chart omissions.** Your documentation should demonstrate the implementation of medical and nursing care plans. If an activity was omitted—for example, a medication not given or a treatment not provided—document the reason for the omission and any actions taken to address the omission, if applicable.

**Co-sign correctly.** Your facility's policy and procedure manual should tell you how to co-sign forms. In many facilities, you'll co-sign doctors' orders to demonstrate that you've read them and have transcribed them on the appropriate charts. This helps ensure that the patient receives prescribed medications and treatments.

**Identify the patient.** To avoid confusion, identify the patient on each page of the clinical record. This helps ensure that you don't chart information on the wrong record and facilitates easy retrieval of patient information.

If you do document information on the wrong clinical record, correct your mistake as described above, according to your facility's policy.

# Documentation and malpractice

Some day, you may find yourself in court as an expert witness (imparting in-depth information on a sub-

ject pertinent to the case), a fact witness (providing details about events surrounding a patient's injury), or even a defendant in a malpractice case. So you should understand some basic information about malpractice and documentation.

Each state has a law defining malpractice, specifying who can be sued under that law. Generally, malpractice occurs when a patient suffers harm as the result of a professional person's wrongful conduct, improper discharge of duties, failure to meet standards of care, or other actions. (See *Leading causes of malpractice suits against nurses,* page 40.)

In a malpractice claim, the patient's lawyer tries to prove that a standard of care wasn't met. Documentation that doesn't offer evidence to the contrary makes the lawyer's job that much easier.

In many malpractice cases, nurses are sued for negligence, a form of malpractice. For a nurse, negligence is defined as the failure to act as a nurse with similar education, experience, and licensure would be expected to act under similar circumstances.

## Four elements of malpractice
If you're charged with malpractice or negligence, the patient's lawyer must prove four elements:
• *Duty.* You must have a legal duty to provide care for the patient and to follow appropriate standards of care.
• *Breach.* You must fail to provide the appropriate care.
• *Damages.* Physical or psychological injury must result from the breach of duty.
• *Proximate cause.* The breach of duty must be the direct cause of the injury.

In *Paavola v. St. Joseph's Hospi-*

## Leading causes of malpractice suits against nurses

The list below shows the most common reasons that malpractice cases are brought against nurses. Remember, to avoid malpractice suits against you and your employer, you must not only provide quality care, but also make sure your documentation indicates that you provided quality care.

**Medication administration**
- Incorrect medications and dosages
- Injury from injections

**Obstetrics and related care**
- Nursing error or negligence causing injury during delivery
- Delay in notifying doctor, causing injury
- Failure to monitor neonate's condition
- Failure to provide proper neonatal care

**Patient falls**
- Side rails left down
- Medicated patients left unattended
- Injury caused when moving or turning patient
- Patient left unattended on stretcher or examination table

**Surgery and related care**
- Foreign object left in patient
- Failure to monitor patient in recovery room
- Negligent postoperative care

**Care involving I.V.s, catheters, and tubes**
- Infiltration
- Negligence causing emboli
- Improper insertion causing injury

**Record keeping**
- Inaccuracy, or failure to record information
- Failure to communicate with doctor
- Breach of confidentiality

**Personal liability**
- Damage to insured's property

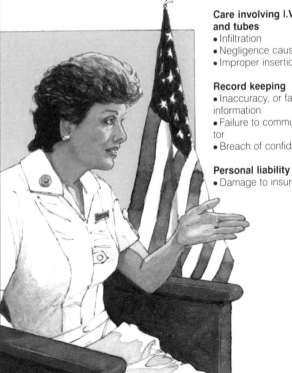

*tal,* the patient's lawyer was able to demonstrate these four elements, and the patient received a $2.1 million settlement. Specifically, the jury decided that the hospital staff — including nurses — failed to identify postsurgical pericardial effusion — a condition that left the patient with brain damage.

In this case, the staff had a duty to monitor the patient for the postoperative complication of pericardial effusion. Their documentation didn't show that they'd monitored him properly; thus, the lawyer demonstrated that they breached their duty. The patient clearly was injured as a result of this breach of duty. Proper monitoring would have meant early detection and treatment. Thus, the proximate cause of the injury was the failure to monitor the patient properly.

As you can see, the key to the patient's case was the lawyer's ability to show that the staff didn't provide proper care. And his evidence was the absence of any documentation showing that the staff monitored the patient properly.

## Suggested readings

*Accreditation Manual for Hospitals.* Chicago: Joint Commission on Accreditation of Healthcare Organizations, 1991.

Bergerson, S.R. "More About Charting With a Jury in Mind," *Nursing88* 18(4):50-58, April 1988.

Claflin, N. "Standards and Quality Assurance," *AACN: Clinical Issues in Critical Care Nursing* 2(1):1-96, February 1991.

Cournoyer, C.P. *The Nurse Manager and the Law.* Rockville, Md.: Aspen Systems Corp., 1989.

Creighton, H. *Law Every Nurse Should Know,* 5th ed. Philadelphia: W.B. Saunders Co., 1986.

Hall, J.K. "Understanding the Fine Line Between Law and Ethics," *Nursing90* 20(10):34-40, October 1990.

Magliozzi, H.M. "Charting That Makes It Through the Medicare Maze," *RN* 53(6):75-79, June 1990.

*Nurse's Handbook of Law and Ethics.* Springhouse, Pa.: Springhouse Corp., 1992.

## Court case citations

Gugino v. Harvard Community Health Plan, 403 N.E. 2d 1966 (Mass. 1980)

Paavola v. St. Joseph's Hospital, 325 N.W. 2d 609 (119 Mich. App. 10, 1982)

Pisel v. Stamford Community Hospital, 180 Conn., 314 (1980)

Villetto v. Weilbaecher, 377 So. 2d 132 (La. Ct. App. 1979)

# 3

# SPECIAL LEGAL SITUATIONS

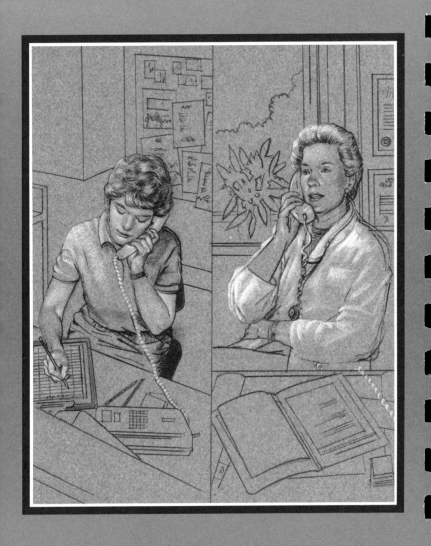

Because of their legal significance, certain situations require special types of documentation. These situations include verifying patient consent, dealing with a patient's refusal of treatment, completing incident reports, witnessing signatures on legal documents, handling living wills, and taking verbal orders. You also have a special legal responsibility to protect the confidentiality of your patient's clinical record when you receive requests for information.

This chapter explains these special situations and reviews your responsibilities. Plus, the chapter gives you guidelines for meeting these responsibilities and avoiding legal pitfalls.

# Patient consent

Required before most treatments and procedures, informed consent means that the patient knows of the proposed therapy and that he agrees to undergo it. A patient verifies this knowledge and consent by signing a consent form.

Legally, the doctor who will perform the treatment or procedure is responsible for obtaining an informed consent. Depending on the policy at your facility, you may be asked to witness the patient's signature.

## Requirements for informed consent

To obtain legally binding informed consent, a doctor must:
• tell the patient of his medical condition and the proposed treatment or procedure. This includes explaining the diagnosis and the nature and purpose of the treatment or procedure, as well as identifying any aspect that's considered experimental.
• describe any risks associated with the treatment or procedure.
• explain the possible consequences of not performing the treatment or procedure.
• describe alternative treatments and procedures, as appropriate.
• tell the patient that he has a right to refuse the treatment or procedure without having other care or support withdrawn. This includes explaining that he can withdraw his consent after giving it.

Also, the patient must agree to the treatment or procedure without any coercion. In fact, if the patient can later prove that he didn't give his consent voluntarily, the procedure could be considered battery. That's because the procedure — a surgery, for instance — would constitute unconsented touching of the patient.

For an informed consent to be valid, the patient must also be legally competent. (See *Who's legally competent?* page 44.)

## Waiving informed consent

The requirements for informed consent can only be waived in two situations. The patient himself may waive them. Or an urgent medical or surgical situation may necessitate a waiver. Many health care facilities have a policy specifying how you should document an emergency that precludes following the guidelines for obtaining an informed consent. Make sure you're familiar with the policy at the facility where you work.

## Witnessing an informed consent signature

Most health care facilities have a standard form that identifies the statutory requirements for informed

## Who's legally competent?

To give informed consent, a person must be legally competent. These two lists show you who's considered competent and who isn't.

**Competent persons**
☐ adults who haven't been declared incompetent
☐ emancipated minors (may include minors who are financially independent or married)
☐ parents or legal guardians of minors
☐ guardians of persons declared legally incompetent
☐ mature minors (status based on factors such as mental status, age, and emotional maturity)

**Incompetent persons**
☐ unemancipated minors and those below the statutory age
☐ patients who've been declared legally incompetent
☐ patients under the influence of narcotics, sedatives, or street drugs

consent. Thus, such a form serves not only as a document to verify a patient's consent but also as a reminder of the requirements for legal consent.

Your health care facility's policy may call for you to witness the patient's signature on an informed consent form. If so, your signature indicates that you saw him sign the consent form and that he was awake, alert, and aware of what he was signing. So if a patient recently received a medication that impairs comprehension (a narcotic, for example), don't have him sign the form. Put it back in the clinical record and notify your supervisor and the attending doctor.

If the patient doesn't understand the doctor's explanation or asks for more information, answer any questions that fall within the scope of your practice. Keep in mind that your legal responsibilities as a witness don't include disclosing all relevant information to the patient. Legally, the doctor has that responsibility; it can't be delegated to you. However, your responsibilities do include documenting your observations in the patient's clinical record and helping the patient get the information he needs from his doctor or other appropriate sources.

Keep in mind that the patient's signature doesn't guarantee informed consent. He could later challenge the validity of the consent in court — claiming, perhaps, that he didn't understand the information he received or that he wasn't given sufficient information to meet the requirements of an informed consent. So even after a patient signs a consent form, if you have doubts about his understanding of his condition or the proposed procedure, consult with the doctor.

Whether you witnessed the signature or not, make sure the patient's clinical record contains the signed consent form before he undergoes the treatment or procedure.

## Refusal of treatment

Any mentally competent adult can legally refuse treatment if he's been fully informed about his medical condition and the likely consequences of his refusal. This patient right stems from the common-law right to be free from unwanted touching and the constitutional rights of religious expression and privacy. Today, courts recognize a competent adult's right to refuse medical treatment even when that refusal will clearly result in his death.

A treatment can be administered after a competent patient has refused it in only one special circumstance — if a doctor or health care facility obtains a court order overruling the patient's decision.

## Documenting a refusal of treatment

When a patient refuses treatment, inform him of the risks involved in making such a decision. If he continues to refuse, notify the doctor, who will then plan the appropriate action. Document the patient's exact words in your progress notes. To cover yourself legally, be sure to document that you didn't provide the prescribed treatment because the patient refused it. Then ask the patient to sign a refusal-of-treatment release form. (See *Using a refusal-of-treatment release form,* page 46.) By indicating that the appropriate treatment would have been given had the patient consented, this form legally protects you, the doctor, and the health care facility.

If the patient refuses to sign the release form, document this refusal in the progress notes. For additional protection, your facility's policy may require you to ask the patient's spouse or closest relative to sign another refusal-of-treatment release form. Document whether or not the spouse or relative does this.

## Discharge against medical advice

The ultimate refusal occurs when a patient seeks a discharge against medical advice (AMA). Although a patient can choose to leave a health

care facility at any time, the law requires clear evidence that he's mentally competent to make that choice. In most facilities, an AMA form serves as a legal document to protect you, the doctors, and the facility should any problems arise from the patient's unapproved discharge. (See *Documenting a discharge against medical advice,* page 47.)

This AMA form should clearly document that the patient knows he's leaving against medical advice, that he's been advised of and understands the risks of leaving, and that he knows he can come back. If a patient refuses to sign the AMA form, document this refusal on the form and enter it in the clinical record. Accurately quote the patient regarding his choice to leave. And make sure you do the following:
• State the patient's reason for leaving AMA.
• Include the names of relatives or others notified of the patient's decision and the dates and times of the notifications.
• Record the risks and consequences of the AMA discharge as explained to the patient and note who explained them.
• Note any instructions regarding alternative sources of follow-up care given to the patient.
• Include a list of those accompanying the patient at discharge and the instructions given to them.
• Note the patient's destination after discharge.

Be sure to document any statements and actions reflecting the patient's mental state at the time he chose to leave the health care facility. This will help protect you, the doctor, and the facility against a charge of negligence. The patient may later claim that his discharge occurred while he was mentally in-

*(Text continues on page 48.)*

**Using a refusal-of-treatment release form**

When a patient refuses treatment, first explain the risks involved in making this choice. Then, if he still refuses to have the treatment, ask him to sign a refusal-of-treatment release form, such as the one below.

---

### REFUSAL-OF-TREATMENT RELEASE FORM

I, _____Jonathan Andrews_____,
(patient's name)

refuse to allow anyone to

_____administer chest PT_____.
(insert treatment)

The risks attendant to my refusal have been fully explained to me, and I fully understand the benefits of this treatment. I also understand that my refusal of treatment seriously reduces my chances for regaining normal health and may endanger my life.

I hereby release

_____Edison Hospital_____,
(name of hospital)

its nurses and employees, together with all doctors in any way connected with me as a patient, from liability for respecting and following my express wishes and direction.

_Dleanie Smith, RN_     _Jonathan Andrews_
(Witness's signature)     (Patient's or legal guardian's signature)

_1/6/92_     _45_
(Date)     (Patient's age)

CHARTING

## Documenting a discharge against medical advice

When a patient wants to leave the hospital against medical advice (AMA), you can encourage him to stay by explaining the risks involved in his decision. If he still wants to leave AMA, document a detailed description of the event in the progress notes and ask him to sign a release form such as the one below.

---

**RESPONSIBILITY RELEASE FORM**

This is to certify that I, _William Roberts_ ,

a patient in _Edison Hospital_ ,
am being discharged against the advice of my doctor and the hospital administration. I acknowledge that I've been informed of the risks involved and hereby release my doctor and the hospital from all responsibility should I suffer any ill effects as a result of this discharge. I also understand that I may return to the hospital at any time and resume treatment.

_William Roberts_
(Patient's signature)

_Joanne Adams, RN_
(Witness's signature)

_1/7/92_
(Date)

_162_
(Patient #)

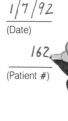
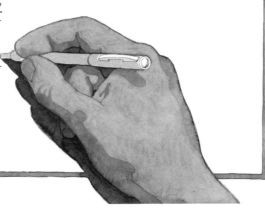

competent and that he wasn't properly supervised while he was in that state.

Also check your facility's policy regarding incident reports. If the patient leaves without anyone's knowledge, or if he refuses to sign the AMA form, you'll probably be required to fill out an incident report.

# Incident reports

The incident report is used to record certain events that are inconsistent with the health care facility's ordinary routine. These include patient injuries, patient complaints, medication errors, and injuries to employees and visitors.

An incident report serves two main purposes. First, it informs the facility's administrators of the incident so changes can be considered to help prevent similar incidents. This is known as risk management. Second, the incident report alerts the administrators and the facility's insurance company to the possibility of a liability claim and the need for further investigation. This is known as claims management.

### Filing an incident report
Only a person with first-hand knowledge of an incident should file a report, and only the person making the report should sign it. Never sign a report describing circumstances or events that you didn't witness personally. Each person with first-hand knowledge should fill out and sign a separate report.

Your report should:
• identify the person involved in the incident.
• document accurately and truthfully

any unusual occurrences that you witnessed.
• record details of what happened and the consequences for the person. Include sufficient information so the administrators can decide whether the matter requires further investigation.
• avoid opinions, judgments, conclusions, or assumptions about who or what caused the incident.
• avoid making suggestions on how to prevent the incident from happening again.

The incident report isn't part of the patient's clinical record, but it may be used in litigation. In general, you shouldn't note in the clinical record that an incident report has been filed. Do, however, include the clinical details of the incident in your progress notes, making sure the descriptions on the incident report and the progress notes mirror each other. (See *Completing an incident report.*)

# Legal documents

Someday, you may be asked to witness a patient's signature on a legal document such as a contract, bill of sale, power of attorney or, more commonly, a will. (See *Witnessing a written will,* page 52.) Before agreeing to do so, consult your health care facility's policy and procedure manual. You may be prohibited from providing this service.

If you do sign as a witness, you're certifying only that you saw a person known to you by a certain name sign the document. You're not attesting to the signer's mental competence — although you shouldn't sign if you question his compe-

*(Text continues on page 52.)*

CHARTING

## Completing an incident report

When you witness a reportable event, you must fill out an incident report. Forms vary among health care facilities, but most include the following information.

---

### INCIDENT REPORT

Name of person

*Mary J. Smith*

Address

*27 Morrison Street, Philadelphia, PA*

| Date of report | Date of incident | Time of incident | If ED patient, give unit number: |
|---|---|---|---|
| 1/9/92 | 1/9/92 | 8:30 a.m. | |

| **LOCATION OF INCIDENT** | **IDENTIFICATION** | |
|---|---|---|
| ☐ patient room | ☑ inpatient | ☐ volunteer |
| ☑ patient bathroom | ☐ ED patient | ☐ visitor |
| ☐ OR | ☐ outpatient | ☐ other _____ |
| ☐ ED | ☐ employee | |
| ☐ hospital grounds | | |
| ☐ nurses' station | Admitting diagnosis of patient | |
| ☐ other _____ | *Diabetes mellitus* | |

| **CONDITION BEFORE INCIDENT** | **Ambulation** | **Side rails** |
|---|---|---|
| **Level of consciousness (previous 4 hours)** | ☑ OOB | ☐ up |
| ☑ alert | ☐ OOB with assistance | ☑ partially up |
| ☐ confused, disoriented | ☐ bed rest with BRP | ☐ down |
| ☐ uncooperative | ☐ complete bed rest | |
| ☐ sedated (drug:_____ ) | ☐ not specified | |
| ☐ unconscious | ☐ other (specify) _____ | |
| | _____ | |

| **Restraints** | **Call system within reach** | **Bed height** |
|---|---|---|
| Present ☐ yes ☑ no | ☑ yes | ☐ high |
| Ordered ☐ yes ☑ no | ☐ no | ☑ low |

| **NATURE OF INCIDENT** | **Medication** | **Surgical** |
|---|---|---|
| **Fall** | ☐ error in patient identification | ☐ consent problem |
| ☐ while ambulatory | ☐ incorrect drug | ☐ incorrect sponge and instrument count |
| ☐ while sitting | ☐ incorrect dosage | |
| ☐ chair    ☐ commode | ☐ incorrect route | ☐ foreign object left in patient |
| ☐ from bed | ☐ timing | ☐ other _____ |
| ☐ off table, stretcher, or equipment | ☐ duplication | |
| ☑ found on floor | ☐ omission | **Burn** |
| ☐ other _____ | ☐ incorrect I.V. solution hung | ☐ chemical |
| | ☐ incorrect I.V. rate | ☐ cigarette |
| | ☐ other _____ | ☐ treatment |
| | | ☐ hot liquid |
| | | ☐ other _____ |

*(continued)*

CHARTING

## Completing an incident report *(continued)*

**NATURE OF INCIDENT** *(continued)*

**Equipment**
Type _____
Control and serial number _____

_____

☐ malfunction
☐ shock
☐ burn
☐ other _____

Date of last maintenance _____
BioMed notified ☐ yes ☐ no
Risk Management notified ☐ yes ☐ no

**Personal property**
☐ damaged
☐ lost
☐ other _____

Describe items.

**Miscellaneous**
☐ patient refuses treatment
☐ needle stick
☐ injuries in treatment
☐ infection
☐ discharge against medical advice
☐ struck by door
☐ other _____

Describe the incident.
*Pt. found sitting on floor in bathroom.*
*Pt. states she slipped.*

_____

**Witnesses:** ☐ yes ☑ no
If yes, note names, addresses, and phone numbers, and indicate if they're
employees, visitors, etc.

1. _____   2. _____

**DISPOSITION**
**Seen by**
☑ attending doctor
☐ ED doctor

**Treatment**
☐ not indicated
☐ treatment given
☐ treatment refused
☑ X-ray ordered
☐ admitted to hospital
☐ follow-up care indicated

Examination findings:
*Tender (L) shoulder*
Doctor's signature:
*John Moyer, MD*

**Notification**
(include your name, the date, and the time)
Attending doctor notified
☑ yes  ☐ no  *Jane Kelley, RN 1/9/92 8:45 a.m.*
Supervisor notified
☑ yes  ☐ no  *Jane Kelley, RN 1/9/92 8:47 a.m.*
Noted in chart
☑ yes  ☐ no  *Jane Kelley, RN 1/9/92 8:49 a.m.*
Sick call request completed
☐ yes  ☑ no

Patient or family notified
☐ yes  ☑ no

☑ Documented in progress notes

CHARTING

## Completing an incident report *(continued)*

---

**GENERAL DATA**
Attending doctor _John W. Moyer, MD_

Room number _439_                Bed number _1_                Shift ☑1 ☐2 ☐3

**Additional details of incident**

_Pt. stated that she slipped on floor_
_when getting out of the shower and hit_
_her ⓛ arm on the door. Pt. complaining_
_of pain in ⓛ shoulder. Pt. escorted_
_back to bed. BP ¹²⁴/₈₀, P 84._
_Dr. Moyer notified @ 8:45 a.m._

---

Signature _Jane Kelly_          Title _RN_          Date _1/9/92_

---

Director's summary (detail follow-up to above incident and action taken)

Signature                    Title                    Date

## Witnessing a written will

When a patient asks you to witness a written will, follow these precautions:
☐ Notify the patient's doctor and your supervisor before you serve as a witness.
☐ Don't give the patient any legal advice.
☐ Don't offer to help him phrase the wording of the document.
☐ Don't comment on the nature of his choices.
☐ Document your actions in your progress notes.

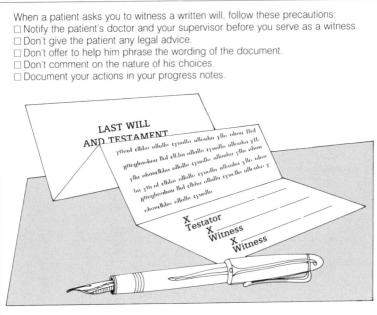

tence — nor are you certifying the presence or absence of duress, undue influence, fraud, or error.

Keep in mind that if you witness a patient's signature on a legal document, you may have to testify that he did indeed sign the document. Expect to answer questions about his mental state when he signed, about any medications or treatments that may have interfered with his ability to make a decision, and about his interactions with family members, his attorney, and others.

### Documenting your role as a witness

When you document in the clinical record that you served as a witness,

specify what type of document was signed, who signed it and when, who was present, and what was done with the document afterward. Also include a description of the patient's mental and physical condition at the time of the signing.

When you witness an oral will or other statement that may have legal significance, record the patient's own words as closely as possible. Also note the names of other witnesses and the patient's physical and mental condition at the time of his statement. Notify the patient's doctor and your supervisor so they know that an item in the patient's clinical record may have legal significance.

# Living wills

In a living will, a legally competent person declares the steps he wants or doesn't want taken in the event of terminal illness. This will doesn't apply to initial treatment decisions—only to those decisions made after a terminally ill patient becomes comatose and has no reasonable possibility of recovery. Typically, a living will authorizes the attending doctor to withhold or discontinue lifesaving procedures. (See *Sample living will,* page 54.)

**Statutory requirements**
Not all states recognize living wills as valid legal instruments. So you should know the laws of your state regarding living wills in case a patient presents you with such a document.

Among states where living wills are accepted, the legal requirements vary. But generally, the laws:
• define the circumstances under which a living will applies.
• indicate the persons authorized to make a living will (usually restricted to competent adults).
• cover any limitations or restrictions as to the care that can be refused. Some statutes don't acknowledge the refusal of food and water.
• describe the elements the will must contain to be considered a legal document, including witnessing requirements.
• identify who's immune from liability for following a living will's directions.
• address the procedures for rescinding a living will.

When a patient presents you with a living will, you should consult your policy and procedure manual for information on how to proceed. And be sure to carefully document the circumstances surrounding the presentation of the document and your handling of the situation.

# Verbal orders

Another area of legal concern is taking and documenting doctors' verbal orders. Errors made interpreting or documenting verbal orders can lead to mistakes in patient care and liability problems for you.

Clearly, verbal orders can be a necessity—especially if you're providing home care. But in a health care facility, you should take verbal orders only in an emergency when the doctor can't immediately attend to the patient.

**Documenting verbal orders**
Carefully follow your facility's policy for documenting a verbal order, using a special form if one exists. Generally, you'll follow this procedure:
• If time and circumstances allow, have another nurse read the order back to the doctor.
• Record the order on the doctor's order sheet as soon as possible. Note the date, then record the order verbatim.
• On the following line, write "v.o." for verbal order or "t.o." for telephone order. Then write the doctor's name and the name of the nurse who read the order back to the doctor.
• Sign your name and write the time.
• Draw lines through any spaces between the order and your verification of the order.

## Sample living will

If your patient has filled out a living will, it may resemble this one. However, the specific wording of your patient's will may differ to reflect both his wishes and the appropriate state statute.

### LIVING WILL DECLARATION

Declaration made this _____ day of _____ 199_____.
I, _____, being of sound mind, willfully and voluntarily make known my desires that my dying shall not be artificially prolonged under the circumstances set forth below, and do declare:

If at any time I should have an incurable injury, disease, or illness certified to be a terminal condition by two (2) doctors who have personally examined me, one of whom shall be my attending doctor, and the doctors have determined that my death will occur whether or not life-sustaining procedures are used and where the application of life-sustaining procedures would serve only to artificially prolong the dying process, I direct that such procedures be withheld or withdrawn and that I be permitted to die naturally with only the administration of medication or the performance of any medical procedure deemed necessary to provide me with comfort or care or to alleviate pain.

In the absence of my ability to give directions regarding the use of such life-sustaining procedures, I want this declaration to be honored by my family and doctor(s) as the final expression of my legal right to refuse medical or surgical treatment and accept the consequences from such refusal.

I understand the full import of this declaration and I am emotionally and mentally competent to make this declaration.

Signed_____ Address_____

I believe the declarant to be of sound mind. I did not sign the declarant's signature above for or at the direction of the declarant. I am at least 18 years of age and am not related to the declarant by blood or marriage, entitled to any portion of the estate of the declarant according to the laws of intestate succession of the _____ or under any will of the declarant or codicil thereto, or directly financially responsible for declarant's medical care. I am not the declarant's attending doctor, an employee of the attending doctor, or an employee of the health care facility in which the declarant is a patient.

Witness _____ Witness _____

Address _____ Address _____

Before me, the undersigned authority, on this _____ day of _____, 199_____, personally appeared _____, and _____, known to me to be the Declarant and the witnesses, respectively, whose names are signed to the foregoing instrument, and who, in the presence of each other, did subscribe their names to the attached declaration (Living Will) on this date, and that said declarant at the time of execution of said declaration was over the age of eighteen (18) years and of sound mind.

(SEAL) Notary Public _____
My commission expires:

Make sure the doctor countersigns the order within the time limits set by your facility's policy. Without this countersignature, you may be held liable for practicing medicine without a license.

# Patient privacy

Your documentation responsibilities also include protecting the confidentiality of the patient's clinical record. Usually, you can't reveal confidential patient information without the patient's permission.

Your patient's legal right to privacy has two bases — the constitutionally implied right of privacy and the common-law statutory right of informational privacy. Besides your legal responsibilities, you also have professional and ethical responsibilities (as specified by the American Nurses' Association, the Joint Commission on Accreditation of Healthcare Organizations, and other professional bodies in their codes and standards) to protect your patient's privacy.

### Ensuring confidentiality

If someone or some agency requests clinical information on a patient, consult your policy and procedure manual for guidance and report the request to your supervisor. If the patient wants to see his record, ask him if he has a question about his treatment you can help him with. Many times, patients ask for their records because they're confused about the care they're receiving. By talking to a patient, you may be able to clear up such confusion.

Be sure you don't release patient records to any unauthorized parties. And don't provide written or oral in-

formation about your patient to anyone, such as visitors or police officers. If you're in doubt as to the validity of a request, notify the doctor and the administrators at the health care facility. Refer all requests from insurance investigators or representatives to the appropriate administrator.

Keep in mind, however, that the law requires you to disclose confidential information in certain situations. These include child abuse cases, matters of public health and safety, and criminal cases. Certain government agencies — for instance, state and local tax bureaus, the Internal Revenue Service, and public health departments — also can order you to reveal confidential information.

But even when circumstances call for some disclosure, be sure to uphold your patient's right to privacy to the greatest extent possible. Consult with your supervisor and follow your facility's policy. And to make doubly sure you don't violate the patient's right to privacy, obtain a written consent from him before disclosing any confidential information to anyone. (See *Who has a right to review the clinical record*, page 56.)

### Keeping computerized records confidential

A computerized system of clinical records dramatically increases the risk of unauthorized access to confidential information. Health care professionals and computer programmers have devised some safeguards to protect patients' privacy. The main safeguard is the signature code.

Through a system of access codes, programmers can limit access to records. For example, your code may allow you to see a patient's entire record, but a technician's code

CHECKLIST

# Who has a right to review the clinical record

Clinical records are the health care facility's property, but the following persons may have a right to see them.

☐ A patient has a right to the information contained in his own record.

☐ Doctors directly involved in a patient's treatment have the right to see his record.

☐ In a lawsuit, the patient's lawyers can secure his record as evidence of the type of care the patient received. The facility's lawyers also may use the record in their defense.

☐ As legal guardians, parents usually have access to their minor children's records and have the right to authorize the release of information to third parties. States can grant a minor control over his record in certain circumstances — for instance, if a minor has a communicable disease, is pregnant, or has a drug or alcohol abuse problem. Some states also guarantee minors the right to privacy if they are high school graduates, are married, or have been pregnant. In most states, persons age 18 and older have the right to privacy, which supersedes their parents' right of access.

☐ The next of kin or the patient's legally authorized representative may seek information when the patient can't assert that right.

☐ The health care facility may allow doctors to review records for research purposes, and the facility may use records for statistical evaluation, research, and education.

☐ Some facilities grant third parties such as insurance companies, lawyers, government agencies, and researchers access to clinical records as long as the patients' anonymity can be protected. Patients should authorize the release first.

☐ Many health insurance companies have agreements with facilities to release certain patient information, as well as agreements with patients allowing access to their information.

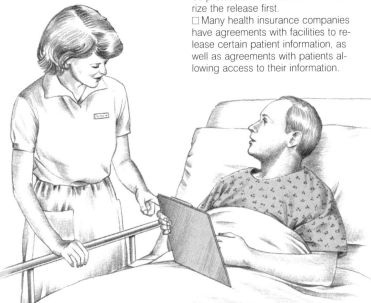

would allow her to see only part of the record. To maximize the effectiveness of such safeguards, never tell anyone your signature code, and promptly notify your supervisor if you suspect someone of using your code.

## Suggested readings

*Accreditation Manual for Hospitals*. Chicago: Joint Commission on Accreditation of Healthcare Organizations, 1991.

Bergerson, S.R. "More About Charting With a Jury in Mind," *Nursing88* 18(4):50-58, April 1988.

Claflin, N. "Standards and Quality Assurance," *AACN: Clinical Issues in Critical Care Nursing* 2(1):1-96, February 1991.

Cournoyer, C.P. *The Nurse Manager and the Law*. Rockville, Md.: Aspen Systems Corp., 1989.

Creighton, H. *Law Every Nurse Should Know,* 5th ed. Philadelphia: W.B. Saunders Co., 1986.

Magliozzi, H.M. "Charting That Makes It Through the Medicare Maze," *RN* 53(6):75-79, June 1990.

*Nurse's Handbook of Law and Ethics*. Springhouse, Pa.: Springhouse Corp., 1992.

Tammelleo, A.D. "Who Can Change a Nurse's Notes?" *RN* 51(5):75-76, May 1988.

# 4

# ASSESSMENT

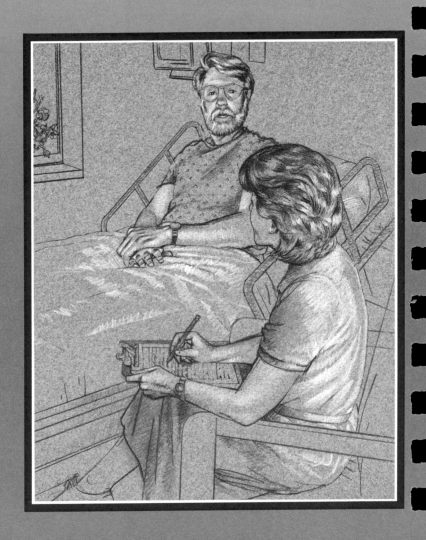

Your assessment of a patient begins when you first encounter him. It continues throughout his hospitalization as you obtain more information about his changing condition. The initial step of the nursing process, assessment includes collecting relevant information from various sources and analyzing it to form a complete picture of your patient.

As you obtain assessment information, you need to document it accurately for several reasons. First of all, accurately recorded assessment information helps guide you through the rest of the nursing process. Using reliable assessment documentation, you can formulate nursing diagnoses, create patient problem lists, and write nursing care plans. Properly documented assessment information also serves as a vital communication tool for other health care team members, forming a baseline from which to evaluate a patient's progress.

You also need to document your assessments accurately to meet the requirements of the Joint Commission on Accreditation of Healthcare Organizations (JCAHO) and various regulatory agencies. And good documentation provides a means to prove that quality care has been given. Peer review organizations and other quality assurance reviewers often look to the nursing assessment data as proof of quality care. Finally, in case of litigation, your record of your assessments can be used as evidence in court.

## Initial assessment

You'll perform your initial assessment when you first meet a patient.

But before getting starting, you should consider two questions:
• What information will be most relevant for this patient?
• How much time do I have to gather the information?
Your answers will help you collect meaningful information during your assessment. This in turn makes comprehensive, goal-directed nursing interventions possible.

### Collecting relevant information
Your initial assessment of a patient may begin with his signs and symptoms, chief complaint, or medical diagnosis. It also may center on the type of care he received in another unit, such as the intensive care unit or the emergency department (ED).

Start by finding out some basic information: Why has the patient sought health care? What are his immediate problems? Are these problems life-threatening? Does a potential for injury exist? What other influences — advanced age, fear, cultural differences, or lack of understanding, for instance — will affect treatment outcomes?

### Complying with the time limit
Your time limit for completing the initial assessment depends on the policy of your health care facility. The JCAHO requires facilities to establish an assessment time limit for each type of patient they serve. Thus, depending on the unit where you work, the time limit may range from 15 minutes to 8 hours.

On medical-surgical units, the initial assessment should usually be completed within 1 hour of the patient's arrival on the unit. Because many facilities offer a wide variety of care, they must establish individual time limits for units or groups of units that share similar patient populations. Thus, a nurse on a trauma

## Clarifying subjective information

To fully explore a patient's complaint, use the PQRST memory device as a guide. When you ask the questions listed here, you'll prompt the patient to describe his symptoms in greater detail. Only when you have such clarifying detail can you properly interpret this subjective information.

| P | Q |
|---|---|
| **PROVOCATIVE OR PALLIATIVE** | **QUALITY OR QUANTITY** |
| • What were you doing when you first experienced or noticed the symptom? What seems to trigger it: stress? position? certain activities? arguments? <br> • What makes the symptom worse? <br> • What relieves the symptom: changing diet? changing position? taking medication? being active? | • How would you describe the symptom — how it feels, looks, or sounds? <br> • How much are you experiencing now? Is it so much that it prevents you from performing any activities? Is it more or less than you experienced at any other time? |

emergency unit or a critical care unit would have a much shorter time limit for completing an initial assessment than a nurse on an elective surgical unit would.

### Categorizing assessment data

When you collect and analyze assessment information, you need to distinguish between two types — subjective and objective. Subjective information represents the patient's perception of his problem. A patient's complaint of chest pain, for example, would be subjective information. Objective information, on the other hand, is something you can observe and verify. A patient's blood pressure reading would be objective information. During your assessment, you'll gather both types of information from primary and secondary sources.

*Subjective data.* The subjective data collected during the patient history generally include the patient's chief complaint or concern, current health status, health history, family history, psychosocial history, activities

| R | S | T |
|---|---|---|
| **REGION OR RADIATION**<br>• Where does the symptom occur?<br>• Does it spread? In the case of pain, does it travel down your back or arms, up your neck, or down your legs? | **SEVERITY SCALE**<br>• How would you rate the symptom at its worst on a scale of 1 to 10, with 10 being the most extreme? Does it force you to lie down, sit down, or slow down?<br>• Does the symptom seem to be getting better, getting worse, or staying about the same? | **TIMING**<br>• On what date did the symptom first occur? What time did it begin?<br>• How did the symptom start: suddenly? gradually?<br>• How often do you experience the symptom: hourly? daily? weekly? monthly?<br>• When do you usually experience it: during the day? at night? in the early morning? Does it awaken you? Does it occur before, during, or after meals? Does it occur seasonally?<br>• How long does an episode of the symptom last? |

of daily living, and review of body systems.

The patient's history, embodying his perception of his problems, is your most important source of assessment information. But it's also subjective, so you must interpret it carefully.

Suppose, for instance, that a patient complains of "frequent stomach pain." To find out what he considers "frequent," ask if the pain occurs once a week, once a day, twice a day, or all day. To find out what he means by "stomach," have

him point to the specific area affected. This will also tell you if the pain is localized or generalized. To find out how he defines "pain," have him describe the sensation. Is it stabbing or dull, twisting or nagging? How does he rate its severity, on a scale of 1 to 10? (See *Clarifying subjective information*.)

When documenting subjective data, be sure to record it as such. Whenever possible, write the patient's own words in quotation marks. And introduce patient statements with a phrase such as "Patient states." For instance, you would document the previous example like this:

Patient states that he has "frequent stomach pain." He describes pain as "dull and nagging." Patient rates pain as a "4" on a scale of 1 to 10. The pain occurs after eating, is relieved by antacids, and is located in the left lower quadrant.

If the patient uses unfamiliar words or phrases, such as slang words, ask him to define them. For clarity, record both the phrase and the patient's definition of it.

*Objective data.* Unlike subjective data, objective data involve no interpretation. If another practitioner were to make the same observations under the same circumstances, she'd obtain the same information. That's why it's important to be specific and avoid using subjective terms, such as "large," "small," or "moderate" when documenting your findings. Whenever possible, use measurements to record data clearly. Specify color, size, and location when appropriate. For instance, "small amount of abdominal wound drainage" could be more clearly described as "about ½ teaspoon of serosanguineous abdominal wound drainage."

Also, avoid interpreting the data and reflecting your opinion. For example, don't write that the "patient is in shock." Instead, document the findings: "pale skin, pulse rate of 140, blood pressure of 90/60 mm Hg."

*Sources of data.* Usually, information gathered directly from the patient—known as primary source data—is the most valuable because it reflects his situation most accu-

rately. Additional data about a patient can be obtained from secondary sources, including family members, friends, and other members of the health care team. Written records—past clinical records, transfer summaries, and personal documents, such as a living will—also provide important information about the patient.

Information from secondary sources often gives you alternative viewpoints to the patient's. And sometimes, because of a patient's condition or age, secondary sources may be essential to establish a complete profile. For example, a child or a patient who's profoundly confused may be able to answer only the simplest questions.

Besides providing essential data, family members and friends give important indications of family dynamics, educational needs, and available support systems. Also, including persons close to the patient helps alleviate their feelings of helplessness during the hospitalization.

### Performing the initial assessment
Your initial assessment consists of your general observations, the health history, and the physical examination.

*General observations.* You can obtain a wealth of information simply by observing the patient. And these observations can begin as soon as you meet him. You may, for instance, observe him while taking him to his room or helping him change into a hospital gown.

You'll continue to make general observations during the interview and physical examination, as well as throughout the patient's hospitalization. By looking critically at the patient, you can collect valuable information about his emotional state, immediate comfort level, and general physical condition. (See *Making general observations,* pages 64 and 65.)

*Maintaining objectivity.* Keep your observations objective and don't draw conclusions. Just document the facts. Remember, initial conclusions are frequently wrong because they're based on too little evidence.

Suppose, for example, that your patient is a middle-aged man who's brought to the ED by ambulance after being found lying in a deserted alley. He appears disheveled, his clothes soiled and torn, with a foul odor of urine and stool. He babbles incoherently, although obscenities are clearly discernible. To document properly, you should record these facts. But you should not conclude that the patient is drunk. He may have diabetes mellitus and be suffering from acute hypoglycemia.

**Health history.** A guide to subsequent physical assessment, the health history organizes pertinent physiologic, psychological, cultural, and psychosocial information. It consists of subjective data about the patient's current health status and provides clues that point to actual or potential health problems. It also reveals the patient's ability to comply with health care interventions and his expectations for treatment outcomes. Finally, the health history yields details about the patient's life-style, family relationships, and cultural influences – all of which may affect his care needs.

Use the health history to identify patient problems that your nursing interventions can help resolve. Your nursing diagnoses then state these problems. And your plan of care is based on your diagnoses.

*Preparing to take the health history.* You'll obtain the patient's health history by interviewing him in a comfortable environment and recording his answers to your questions. If appropriate, also interview the patient's family members and close friends.

Before the interview, consider the patient's ability and readiness to participate. For example, if he's sedated or confused, hostile or angry, or if he's experiencing pain or dyspnea, ask only the most essential questions. You can perform a more in-depth interview later, when his condition improves. In the meantime, secondary sources can often provide much of the needed information.

Try to alleviate as much of the patient's discomfort and anxiety as possible. Also attempt to create a quiet, private environment for your talk. Avoid interruptions by arranging for another nurse to cover your other patients during the interview. Your efforts let your patient know you're interested in what he tells you, and that you respect the confidentiality of the information he shares. (See *Creating a comfortable interview setting,* pages 66 and 67.)

Tell the patient how long the interview will last – usually from 15 to 30 minutes for a medical-surgical patient. Explain the purpose of the history so he understands why you'll be asking him personal questions. Finally, be calm, relaxed, and unhurried. Your actions will convey to the patient the importance of the health history interview.

*Conducting the interview.* You need to show empathy, compassion, self-awareness, and objectivity to promote a trusting relationship with your patient – the first step toward a successful interview. To obtain a

comprehensive health history, you'll
also need to use a variety of interviewing techniques. Here are some
examples:

• *Using general leads.* Broad open-
ing questions allow the patient to
relate information that he deems essential. Asking something such as
"What brought you to the hospital?"
or "What concerns do you have?"
encourages the patient to discuss
what's most important to him.

• *Restating (summarizing) information.* To help clarify the patient's
meaning, restate the essence of his
comments. For instance, suppose a
patient says, "I have pain after I eat"
and you respond, "So, you have
pain about three times a day." This
might prompt the patient to reply,
"Oh no, I only eat breakfast and
then the pain is so severe that I
don't eat for the rest of the day."

• *Using reflection.* Asking a question
in a different way offers the patient
an opportunity to reconsider his response. A patient might state, "I've
told you everything about my home
life." Using reflection, you might respond, "Do you have any other concerns about your situation after you
leave the hospital?"

• *Stating the implied meaning.* A patient may hint at difficulties or problems. By stating what has been
unspoken, you give him an opportunity to clarify his thoughts and accurately interpret the meaning of
his statements. A patient who re-
marks, "I'm sure my wife is glad
that I'm in the hospital" may be im-
plying several things. To clarify this
statement, you might respond, "By
saying your wife is glad, do you
mean she's been concerned about
your condition, or do you feel
you've been a burden to her at
home?"

• *Focusing the discussion.* Patients
often stray from the topic at hand to

## Making general observations

Your general observations of the patient's appearance, cognitive functions, communication ability, and
mobility form an important part of your
initial assessment. These lists give you
the specific characteristics to look for
and to document.

### Appearance
*Age*
☐ Appears to be stated age
☐ Appears older or younger than
stated age
*Physical condition*
☐ Physically fit, strong, and appropri-
ate weight for height
☐ Out of shape, weak, and either un-
derweight or overweight
☐ Apparent limitations, such as an
amputation or paralysis
☐ Obvious scars, rash
*Dress*
☐ Dressed appropriately or inappro-
priately for season
☐ Clean and well-kept clothes
☐ Clothes soiled or torn; smell of alco-
hol, urine, or feces
*Personal hygiene*
☐ Clean and well-groomed
☐ Unkempt; dirty skin, hair, and nails;
unshaved
☐ Body odor or unusual breath odor
*Skin color*
☐ Pale, ruddy, cyanotic, jaundiced, or
tanned

### Cognitive functions
*Awareness*
☐ Oriented; aware of surroundings
☐ Disoriented; unaware of person,
place, time
*Mood*
☐ Responds appropriately; talkative
☐ Answers in one-word responses; of-
fers information only in response to di-
rect questions
☐ Hesitant to answer questions; looks
to family member before answering

□ Angry; states "Leave me alone" (or similar response); speaks loudly and abruptly to family members
□ Maintains, or avoids, eye contact
*Thought processes*
□ Maintains a conversation; makes relevant statements; follows commands appropriately
□ Mind seems to wander; makes irrelevant statements; follows commands inappropriately

## Communication
*Speech*
□ Speaks clearly in English or other language
□ Speaks only with one-word responses; doesn't respond to verbal stimuli
□ Speech seems slurred, hoarse, loud, soft, incoherent, hesitant, slow, fast, or nonsensical
□ Has difficulty completing sentences due to shortness of breath or pain
*Hearing*
□ Hears well enough to respond to questions
□ Hard of hearing; wears hearing aid; must speak loudly into left or right ear
□ Deaf; reads lips or uses sign language
*Vision*
□ Sees well enough to read instructions in English or other language
□ Wears glasses to see or to read
□ Can't read
□ Blind

## Mobility
*Ambulation*
□ Walks independently; steady gait
□ Uses a cane, crutches, walker
□ Unsteady, slow, hesitant, or shuffling gait; leans toward one side; can't support own weight
□ Transfers from chair to bed independently
□ Needs assistance (from one, two, or three people) to transfer from chair to bed
*Movement*
□ Moves all extremities
□ Has right- or left-sided weakness; paralysis
□ Can't turn in bed independently
□ Has jerky or spastic movements of body parts (specify)

## Creating a comfortable interview setting

To create an interview setting in which your patient feels comfortable enough to share confidential information, use the following tips:

☐ *Maintain privacy.* If the patient is in a semi-private room but he's ambulatory, take him to a quiet area outside the room. If he isn't ambulatory but his roommate is, you might ask the roommate to leave you alone with the patient for the length of time you'll need for the interview. If you can't achieve privacy with your patient in or outside his room, draw the curtains around

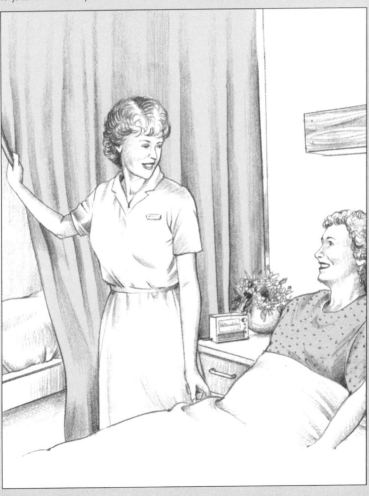

the bed and speak in a low tone to convey respect for his privacy.

□ *Reduce noise.* Noise in the immediate environment distracts both you and the patient. If a television or radio is on in the room, ask the patient if you may turn it off or lower the volume. If the corridor or neighboring rooms are noisy and you can't move the patient to a quiet area, ask the noisy persons to keep their voices down. Then close the patient's door.

□ *Eliminate odors.* Try to remove all unpleasant odors from the immediate area before the interview. Be sure to allow enough time for the odor from spray disinfectants to dissipate.

□ *Adjust the lighting.* If the room is too dark, you may have trouble maintaining eye contact with your patient and observing his gestures and facial expressions. If the room is too bright, the patient may feel that he's being interrogated. Also, eye fatigue may result. Indirect, moderate lighting works best. Before you change the lighting, ask the patient's permission to do so. Explain why you want to change the lighting, too. For example, you might say something such as "I'd like to adjust the shades because the sunlight is causing a glare in your room. Is that all right with you?"

□ *Maintain a comfortable temperature.* If the room is too warm or too cool, have the temperature adjusted (if possible), after asking the patient's permission. Or provide the patient with extra blankets or ventilation as necessary. Maintain the room temperature between 65° and 72° F (18.3° and 22.2° C).

□ *Use appropriate body language.* Sit down to conduct the interview. Studies show that this often makes the interview last longer, while also letting your patient know you care about what he tells you.

relate other information they feel you should know. You need to get the conversation back on track without insulting the patient or making him feel that the information isn't important. To help a patient refocus the conversation, you might say something such as "That's very interesting, but first I'd like to get back to our discussion about your last hospitalization."

• *Asking open-ended questions.* Questions that encourage the patient to express himself elicit more information than questions that call for a one-word response. If you ask, "Do you take your medications?" the patient may respond with a simple "Yes." But if you ask, "How do you take your medications?" you might discover that the patient takes his antihypertensive pills sporadically because they make him feel dizzy.

To avoid alienating the patient during the interview and thus hindering communication, don't use the following techniques:

• *Judgmental or threatening questions.* A patient shouldn't have to justify his feelings or actions. Questions such as "Why did you do that?" or demanding statements such as "Explain your behavior" may be perceived as a threat or challenge. They force the patient to defend himself. What's more, when a patient doesn't have a specific answer to this type of question, he may tend to invent an appropriate response, merely to satisfy you.

• *Probing and persistent questions.* This style of questioning can make the patient feel manipulated and defensive. Make only one or two attempts to obtain information about a particular subject. If the patient seems to be avoiding the topic or is hesitant to answer, reevaluate the relevance of the information. Re-

spect the patient's right to privacy.
• *Inappropriate language.* Don't use technical terms or jargon when interviewing the patient. Questions such as "Do you take that med q.i.d. or p.r.n.?" can intimidate or alienate the patient and his family. Using unfamiliar language can make the patient feel you're unwilling to share information about his condition or to converse on his level.
• *Advice.* Giving advice implies that you know what's best for the patient. Instead, you should encourage the patient and family members to participate in health care decisions. If the patient asks for advice, help him explore his own opinions about the available options.
• *False reassurances.* Statements such as "You'll be all right" or "Everything will work out fine" tend to devalue a person's feelings. By recognizing those feelings, you can open communication channels. Saying something such as "You seem worried or frightened" encourages the patient to speak candidly. Always try to be honest and sensitive. Even when a patient asks, "Am I going to die?" you can honestly state, "I don't know. Tell me what makes you ask that."

*Timesaving measures.* Increased patient acuity and staff shortages sometimes make it difficult to conduct a thorough patient interview. But certain strategies can help you make the most of the time you have without compromising quality. (See *Making the most of your interview time.*)

In certain circumstances, you may not have to conduct a patient interview. Instead, you can have the patient complete a questionnaire about his past and present health status. Then you can quickly and easily document his health history by re-

viewing the information on the questionnaire. This method has been most successful in short procedures units and before admission for elective procedures. Although it saves time, this method doesn't give you an opportunity to develop a positive relationship with your patient.

**Physical examination.** You'll perform the physical examination by using the assessment techniques of inspection, palpation, percussion, and auscultation. During this phase of the assessment, you'll obtain objective data that may confirm or rule out suspicions raised during the health history interview. Your findings will enable you to plan care and start teaching your patient about his condition. For example, an elevated blood pressure reading tells you that a patient may need a sodium-restricted diet and, possibly, patient teaching on how to control hypertension.

The scope of the physical examination depends on the patient's condition, the clinical setting, and the policies and procedures established by your health care facility. A routine neurologic examination on a medical-surgical unit, for example, may include assessing level of consciousness, orientation, muscle strength, and pupillary response. Abnormal findings would then call for you to perform a more in-depth assessment — an assessment that would be routine on a neurologic unit or critical care unit.

The major components of the physical examination include height, weight, vital signs, and a review of the major body systems. A routine review of systems for an adult patient on a medical-surgical unit includes the following.

*Respiratory system.* Note the rate

and rhythm of respirations, and auscultate the lung fields. Inspect the lips, mucous membranes, and nail beds. Also inspect any sputum, noting color, consistency, and other characteristics.

*Cardiovascular system.* Note the color and temperature of the extremities and assess the peripheral pulses. Also check for edema and note hair growth on the extremities. Inspect the neck veins and auscultate heart sounds.

*Neurologic system.* Inspect the patient's head for evidence of trauma. Then, assess his level of consciousness, noting his orientation to person, place, and time, and his ability to follow commands. Also assess his pupillary reactions. Check his extremities for movement and sensation.

*Eyes, ears, nose, and throat.* Assess the patient's ability to see objects with or without corrective lenses, as appropriate. Also assess his ability to hear spoken words clearly. Inspect the eyes and ears for discharge; the nasal mucous membranes for dryness, irritation, and the presence of blood; and the teeth for cleanliness. If appropriate, note how well the patient's dentures fit. Observe the condition of the oral mucous membranes, and palpate the lymph nodes in the neck.

*GI system.* Auscultate for bowel sounds in all quadrants. Note the presence of abdominal distention or ascites, and assess the condition of mucous membranes around the anus.

*Musculoskeletal system.* Assess the range of motion of major joints. Look for any swelling at the joints,

TIMESAVING TIP

## Making the most of your interview time

When you're pressed for time, the following tips will help you obtain a health history more quickly:
• Before the interview, fill in as much of the health history information as you can from secondary sources, such as admission forms, transfer summaries, and the medical history. This avoids duplication of effort and reduces interview time. If some of this information needs clarification, you can ask the patient to give you a fuller explanation. For instance, you might say something such as "You told Dr. Smith that you have periodic dizzy spells. Do you think you could tell me more about those spells?"
• Check your facility's policy regarding who can gather assessment data. You may be able to have a nursing assistant or an LPN collect routine information, such as allergies and past hospitalizations. Remember, however, you must review the information and verify it as necessary.
• Begin by asking about the patient's chief complaint and the reason for his hospitalization. Then, if the interview is interrupted; you'll have some initial information on which to base a care plan.
• Use your facility's nursing assessment documentation form only as a guide to organize information. Ask your patient only pertinent questions from the form.
• Take only brief notes during the interview. That way, your note taking won't interrupt the flow of conversation. Complete longer summations or expand on information as soon as possible after you complete the interview. You can always go back to the patient if you need to clarify or verify information.
• Record your findings in concise, specific phrases. Use approved abbreviations.

as well as for any contractures, muscular atrophy, or obvious deformity.

*Genitourinary system.* Note any bladder distention or incontinence. If indicated, inspect the genitalia for rashes, edema, or deformity. (Inspection of the genitalia may be waived at the patient's request or if no dysfunction was reported during the interview.)

*Reproductive system.* If indicated, inspect the genitalia for sexual maturity. Also examine the breasts, noting any abnormalities.

*Integumentary system.* Note any sores, lesions, scars, decubiti, rashes, bruises, or petechia. Also note the patient's skin turgor.

# Meeting JCAHO requirements

The JCAHO requires that health care professionals in accredited facilities meet certain standards for performing patient assessments. By reviewing the documentation of patient assessments, the JCAHO determines whether these standards have been met.

One key JCAHO requirement is that you obtain assessment information from the patient's family or friends, when appropriate. When you interview someone close to the patient who isn't part of his family, make sure you note the nature of the relationship and the length of time the person has known the patient. For instance, in your documentation, you might write something such as "Information

supplied by Daniel Rosenberger, a friend who has lived with the patient for 3 years."

**Assessment requirements**
Current JCAHO standards mandate that each patient's initial assessment includes six elements: biophysical factors, psychosocial factors, environmental factors, self-care capabilities, learning needs, and discharge planning needs.

*Biophysical factors.* These include physical examination findings from your review of the major body systems.

*Psychosocial factors.* These include the patient's fears, anxieties, and other concerns related to his hospitalization. To find out what support systems the patient has, you might ask something such as "How does being in the hospital affect your home situation?" or "How is your family coping while you're hospitalized?" A patient's concerns about these matters may impair his willingness or ability to comply with health care interventions.

*Environmental factors.* The patient's home environment affects his need for care both during hospitalization and after discharge. Ask where he lives, and whether he lives in a house or an apartment. Does his home have adequate heat, ventilation, hot water, and bathroom facilities? How many flights of stairs does he have to climb? Does the layout of the home pose any hazards?

Ask if his home is near a shopping area. How far does he have to travel to visit a doctor or health care facility? Does he use special equipment at home for activities of daily living that isn't available in the hospital?

CHECKLIST

## Discharge assessment: Identifying potential problems

When you're assessing your patient, note whether any of the following descriptions fit him. If so, he may need extra help after discharge.
☐ Copes poorly with chronic illness or permanent disability
☐ Frequently readmitted within a short time for same condition (two or more times a year)
☐ Acutely ill with poor prognosis
☐ Newly diagnosed with chronic or terminal illness
☐ Age 70 or older
☐ Suspected or confirmed victim of abuse or neglect

☐ Possible substance abuser
☐ Suspected of being unable or unwilling to comply with treatments
☐ Has no family
☐ Has family that can't meet discharge needs
☐ Has insurance that doesn't cover care needs after discharge
☐ Unable to function without community services or resources
☐ Lives a considerable distance from health care facility
☐ Lives in residence that's unsanitary or in poor condition
☐ Has no known address

Tailor your questions to the patient's condition and the geographic setting of the health care facility.

***Self-care capabilities.*** A patient's ability to perform activities of daily living affects how well he complies with his therapy both before and after discharge. So you must assess your patient's ability to eat, wash, use the bathroom, turn in bed, get out of bed, and get around. At some health care facilities, you'll use a checklist to indicate if a patient can perform these tasks independently or if he needs partial or total assistance.

***Learning needs.*** An early assessment of what the patient needs to know about his condition leads to effective patient teaching. During the initial assessment, you should evaluate your patient's knowledge of the disease process, self-care, diet, medications, life-style changes, treatment measures, and any limitations resulting from the disease or its treatment.

One way to evaluate your patient's educational needs is to ask open-ended questions, such as "What do you know about the medicine you take?" His response will tell you if he understands and complies with his medication regimen, or if he needs more teaching.

You should also assess factors that may hinder learning. These include the nature of the patient's illness or injury, as well as his health beliefs, religious beliefs, educational level, sensory deficits (such as hearing difficulties), language barriers, stress level, age, and any pain or discomfort he may be experiencing.

***Discharge planning needs.*** As with patient teaching, discharge planning should begin as soon as possible. You must identify the discharge planning needs of every patient — especially those who are most likely to require help after discharge. (See *Discharge assessment: Identifying potential problems.*)

Find out where the patient will go after discharge. Will follow-up care be accessible? Are community resources, such as visiting nurse services and Meals on Wheels, available where the patient lives? Answers to such questions help you to plan effectively for your patient's discharge.

# Documenting the initial assessment

Depending on where you work, you may hear the initial assessment information referred to by any of several names, including the "nursing admission assessment" and the "nursing data base." Documentation styles and formats also vary, depending on the facility's policy and the patient population. What's more, health care facilities have different policies for documenting learning needs, discharge planning, and incomplete initial assessment data. So you must be familiar with your facility's standards to document your initial assessment findings appropriately.

## Documentation styles
Initial assessment findings are documented in one of three basic styles: narrative note, standardized open-ended style, and standardized close-ended style. Many assessment forms use a combination of all three styles.

***Narrative note.*** This consists of a handwritten account in paragraph form, summarizing information obtained by general observation, interview, and physical examination.

While narrative notes allow you to list your findings in order of importance, they also pose problems. Frequently, the notes mimic the medical model by focusing on a review of body systems. They're also time-consuming — both to write and to read. Plus, narrative notes require you to remember and record all significant information in a detailed, logical sequence — often an unrealistic goal in today's hectic world of health care. Finally, difficulty in interpreting handwriting can easily lead to a misinterpretation of findings.

Narrative notes are most practical for independent practitioners and home care or community nurses. Within health care institutions, however, exclusive use of narrative notes wastes time and may jeopardize quality assurance.

***Standardized open-ended style.*** The typical "fill-in-the blanks" assessment form comes with preprinted headings and questions. This form saves you time in a couple of ways. Information is categorized under specific headings, so you can easily record and retrieve it. And the form can be completed using partial phrases and approved abbreviations. (See *Completing a standardized open-ended form.*)

Unfortunately, however, open-ended forms don't always provide the space or the instructions to encourage thorough descriptions. Thus, following the heading *type of dwelling,* one nurse may write "apartment" whereas another may write "apartment with four-flight walk-up, without heat or hot water."

Nonspecific responses can, of course, lead to misinterpretation. For instance, a nurse may write that a patient performs a certain task "within normal limits." But unless normal limits have been defined, this notation is neither clear nor legally sound.

CHARTING

## Completing a standardized open-ended form

At some health care facilities, you may use a standardized open-ended form to document initial assessment information. Below you'll find a portion of such a form.

**Reason for hospitalization** "*fell in bathroom*," "*broke hip*"

**Expected outcomes** *By discharge, pt. and family will describe position and activity recommendations and restrictions, demonstrate care of injury site, and identify signs and symptoms of hip injury complications.*

**Last hospitalization**

Date *1/83* Reason *high blood pressure*

**Medical history** *hypertension, diabetes mellitus*

**Medications and allergies**

| Drug | Dosage | Time of last dose | Patient's statement of drug's purpose |
|------|--------|-------------------|---------------------------------------|
| *Humulin N* | *30 units b.i.d.* | *7:30 a.m.* | "*for sugar*" |
| *Lasix* | *10 mg q. daily* | *10:00 a.m.* | "*water pill*" |
| *Minipress* | *1 mg t.i.d.* | *8:00 a.m.* | "*for BP*" |

| Allergy | Reaction |
|---------|----------|
| *shellfish* | "*hives*" |

***Standardized close-ended style.*** This type of assessment form provides preprinted headings, checklists, and questions with specific responses. You simply check off the appropriate response. (See *Completing a standardized close-ended form*, page 74.)

Besides saving time, the close-ended form eliminates the problem of illegible handwriting and makes checking documented information easy. Plus, the form can be easily incorporated into most computerized systems. The form also clearly establishes the type and amount of information required by the facility. And even though the forms often

## Completing a standardized close-ended form

At some health care facilities, you may use a standardized close-ended form to document initial assessment information. Below you'll find a portion of such a form.

### SELF-CARE ABILITY

| Activity | 1 | 2 | 3 | 4 | 5 | 6 |
|---|---|---|---|---|---|---|
| Bathing | | | ✓ | | | |
| Cleaning | | | ✓ | | | |
| Climbing stairs | | | ✓ | | | |
| Cooking | | | ✓ | | | |
| Dressing and grooming | | | ✓ | | | |
| Eating and drinking | ✓ | | | | | |
| Moving in bed | ✓ | | | | | |
| Shopping | | | ✓ | | | |
| Toileting | | | | ✓ | | |
| Transferring | | | ✓ | | | |
| Walking | | | ✓ | | | |
| Other home functions | | | ✓ | | | |

**Key**
1 Independent
2 Requires assistive device
3 Requires personal assistance
4 Requires personal assistance and assistive device
5 Dependent
6 Experienced change in last week

**ASSISTIVE DEVICES**
☑ Bedside commode
☐ Brace or splint
☐ Cane
☐ Crutches
☐ Feeding device
☐ Trapeze
☐ Walker
☐ Wheelchair
☐ Other
☐ None

**ACTIVITY TOLERANCE**
☐ Normal
☑ Weakness
☐ Dizziness
☐ Exertional dyspnea
☐ Dyspnea at rest
☐ Angina
☐ Pain at rest
☐ Oxygen needed
☐ Intermittent claudication
☐ Unsteady gait
☐ Other

**REST PATTERN**
**Sleep habits**
☑ Less than 8 hours
☐ 8 hours
☐ More than 8 hours
☐ Morning nap
☑ Afternoon nap
**Sleep difficulties**
☐ Insomnia
☑ Early awakening
☐ Unrefreshing sleep
☐ Nightmares
☐ None

use nonspecific terminology, such as "within normal limits" or "no alteration," guidelines clearly define these responses.

The close-ended form also creates some problems. For instance, many of these forms provide no place to record relevant information that doesn't fit the preprinted choices. And the forms tend to be lengthy,

especially when a hospital's policy calls for recording in-depth physical assessment data.

### Documentation formats
Historically, nursing assessment has followed a medical format, emphasizing the patient's initial symptoms and a comprehensive review of body systems. (See *A medical model for*

CHARTING

## A medical model for nursing assessment

At some health care facilities, nursing assessment forms are still based on the medical model. The physical examination section of this form is organized according to a comprehensive review of body systems.

**SYSTEMS REVIEW**

Admission date and time: _12/11/91    10:00 a.m._

Height: _5' 5"_ Weight: _140_ TPR: _98⁶    88    22_

BP, right arm: _132/94_ BP, left arm: _132/94_

Check boxes or write descriptions as appropriate.

**Mental status**
☑ Alert
☑ Cooperative
☐ Calm
☐ Lethargic
☐ Withdrawn
☐ Depressed
☐ Agitated
☑ Anxious
Oriented to:
☑ Time
☑ Place
☑ Person

**Speech**
☑ Normal, clear
☐ Slurred
☐ Hesitant
☐ Hoarse
☐ Dysphasic

**Neurologic system**
☑ Normal
☑ Pupils: PERRLA
☐ Dizziness
☐ Headaches
☐ Numbness
☐ Paraplegia
☐ Hemiplegia, right
☐ Hemiplegia, left
Comments:_____
_____
_____

**Eyes**
☐ Normal
☐ Glasses
☑ Contact lenses
☐ Implanted lenses
☐ Blind, right eye
☐ Blind, left eye
☐ Artificial prosthesis
☐ Discharge
☐ Diplopia
☐ Blurred vision
☐ Tearing
☐ Burning
☐ Itching
☐ Photophobia
☐ Pain
☐ Sclera color _____
☐ Cataract
☐ Glaucoma

**Ears**
☐ Normal
☐ Hearing loss
☐ Hearing aid
☑ Tinnitus
☐ Vertigo
☐ Discharge
☐ Pain

**Nose**
☐ Normal
☑ Sinusitis
☐ Rhinitis
☐ Discharge
☐ Obstruction
☐ Epistaxis

**Mouth and throat**
☐ Normal
☑ Dentures, upper
☑ Dentures, lower
☐ Partial plate
☐ Dental fillings
☐ Sores on tongue
☐ Gum swelling or
bleeding
☐ Diminished taste
☐ Sore throat

**Respiratory system**
☐ Normal
☑ Dyspnea
☑ Cough
☐ Hemoptysis
☐ Pain
☐ Orthopnea
☑ Breath sounds _crackles, posterior lobes_

**Cardiovascular system**
☐ Normal
☑ Edema
☐ Cyanosis
☐ Cold extremities
☐ Palpitations
Pulse:
☑ Regular
☐ Irregular
☐ Bounding
☐ Weak
☑ Thready
☑ Pedal pulse, right _palpable_
☑ Pedal pulse, left _palpable_
☑ Heart sounds
_S₄ c̄ summation gallop_

CHARTING

## A medical model for nursing assessment *(continued)*

### SYSTEMS REVIEW *(continued)*

**GI system**
- ☐ Normal
- ☐ Change in appetite
- ☐ Indigestion
- ☐ Flatulence
- ☐ Nausea
- ☐ Vomiting
- ☐ Bleeding
- ☐ Abdominal pain
- ☐ Abdominal distention
- ☐ Ascites
- ☐ Hemorrhoids
- ☐ Constipation
- ☐ Diarrhea
- ☑ Last bowel movement *12/10/91*
- ☑ Number of stools per day *2*
- Bowel sounds:
- ☑ Present
- ☐ Absent
- ☐ Hyperactive
- ☐ Other: _____

**Nutritional status**
- ☐ Special diet *N/A*
- ☑ Recent weight gain
- ☐ Recent weight loss

**GU system**
- ☑ Normal
- ☐ Frequency
- ☐ Urgency
- ☐ Dysuria
- ☐ Nocturia
- Number of times _____
- ☐ Bleeding
- ☐ Burning
- Comments: _____

**Reproductive system—female**
- ☑ Last menstrual period *1988*
- ☐ Cramping
- ☐ Irregular bleeding
- ☐ Discharge
- ☐ Vaginal infections
- ☐ Pain or difficulty with intercourse
- ☑ Menopause
- ☐ Other: _____

**Reproductive system—male**
- ☐ Prostate problems
- ☐ Lesions
- ☐ Impotence
- ☐ Other: _____

**Musculoskeletal system**
- ☐ Normal
- ☐ Stiffness
- ☐ Pain
- ☐ Weakness
- ☐ Limited ROM
- ☐ Paralysis
- ☐ Tenderness
- ☐ Swelling
- ☑ Arthritis
- ☐ Prosthesis
- ☐ Other: _____
- Physical activity:
- ☑ No limitations
- ☐ Walks with help
- ☐ Uses cane
- ☐ Uses crutches
- ☐ Uses walker
- ☐ Bedridden

**Skin**
- ☐ Turgor _____
- ☑ Temperature *cool*
- ☑ Color *pale*
- ☐ Dry
- ☐ Moist
- ☑ Diaphoretic
- ☐ Rash
- ☐ Eczema
- ☐ Acne
- ☐ Bruises
- ☐ Burns
- ☐ Lumps
- ☐ Lacerations
- ☐ Abrasions
- ☐ Scars _____
- ☐ Other: _____
- Condition of:
- ☑ Hair *clean and neat*
- ☑ Nails *clean*
- Pressure ulcers *none*
- ☐ Number _____
- ☐ Stage 1, 2, 3, 4
- ☐ Location _____
- ☐ Describe _____

Additional comments:

_____

_____

Date and time completed  *12 / 11 / 91   10:30 a.m.*

RN signature  *Mary Peckett, RN*

*nursing assessment,* pages 75 and 76.) Although many health care facilities still use a medical format to organize their nursing assessment forms, some facilities have adopted formats that more readily reflect the nursing process.

Most facilities that use a nursing format for assessment base it on either human response patterns or functional health care patterns. Other documentation formats are modeled on specific conceptual frameworks based on published nursing theories.

***Human response patterns.*** As you know, the North American Nursing Diagnosis Association (NANDA) has developed a classification system for nursing diagnoses based on human response patterns. These patterns relate directly to actual or potential health problems as indicated by assessment data.

Thus, when you use an assessment form organized by these patterns, you can easily establish appropriate diagnoses while you record assessment data — especially if a listing of diagnoses is included with the form. The main drawback is that these forms tend to be lengthy. (See *Human response patterns,* page 78 and *Documenting human response patterns,* page 79.)

***Functional health care patterns.*** Some health care facilities organize their assessment data according to functional health care patterns. Developed by Marjory Gordon, this system classifies nursing data according to the patient's ability to function independently. (See *Functional health care patterns,* page 80 and *Documenting functional health care patterns,* page 81.)

Many nurses consider functional health care patterns easier to understand and remember than human response patterns. Generally, assessment forms based on functional health care patterns are easier and less time-consuming to complete.

***Conceptual frameworks.*** At some health care facilities, assessment forms have been modeled on the nursing philosophies that the nursing departments follow. Some examples include Dorothea Orem's self-care model, Imogene King's theory of goal attainment, and Sister Callista Roy's adaptation model. Assessment forms based on these nursing philosophies reflect the individual theory's approach to nursing care.

## Documenting learning needs

Most initial assessment forms have a separate section for documenting a patient's learning needs. When you reassess your patient's learning needs, you can document your findings in the progress notes, on an open-ended patient education flow sheet, or on a structured patient education flow sheet designed for a specific problem, such as diabetes mellitus.

## Documenting discharge planning needs

Effective discharge planning begins when you identify and document the patient's needs during the initial assessment. Depending on the policy at your health care facility, you'll record the patient's discharge needs on the initial assessment form (in a designated section), on a specially designed discharge planning form, in a separate section on the patient care card file, in the progress notes, or on a discharge planning flow sheet. (See *Documenting discharge planning,* page 82.)

# Human response patterns

This list gives you the nine human response patterns along with their definitions. Following each definition, you'll find the areas you need to assess.

**Exchanging**
This pattern involves mutual giving and receiving.
☐ Nutrition
☐ Body temperature
☐ Infection
☐ Bowel elimination
☐ Urine elimination
☐ Fluid balance
☐ Tissue perfusion
☐ Gas exchange
☐ Airway patency
☐ Skin and tissue integrity
☐ Potential for injury

**Communicating**
This pattern involves sending messages.
☐ Speech abilities
☐ Language usage

**Relating**
This pattern involves establishing bonds with other people.
☐ Social interactions
☐ Family dynamics
☐ Role performance
☐ Sexuality

**Valuing**
This pattern involves assigning relative worth to other people, objects, and concepts.
☐ Spirituality
☐ Cultural influences

**Choosing**
This pattern involves selecting alternatives.
☐ Coping mechanisms
☐ Compliance with health promotion activities

**Moving**
This pattern involves activity.
☐ Usual activity levels
☐ Ambulation
☐ Overall movement capabilities
☐ Sleep patterns
☐ Diversional activities
☐ Self-care abilities
☐ Home care management

**Perceiving**
This pattern involves receiving information.
☐ Sensory abilities
☐ Self-concept
☐ Body image

**Knowing**
This pattern involves the meaning associated with information.
☐ Thought processes
☐ Learning needs

**Feeling**
This pattern involves the subjective awareness of information.
☐ Pain
☐ Discomfort
☐ Fear, anxieties
☐ Grief
☐ Violent behavior toward self or others

## Documenting incomplete initial data

No matter which assessment tool you use, you may not always be able to obtain a complete health history during the initial assessment. For instance, the patient may be too ill to participate, and secondary sources may be unavailable.

*(Text continues on page 83.)*

CHARTING

## Documenting human response patterns

Below you'll find one page of an assessment form that's organized by human response patterns. The sequence of response patterns varies among forms.

### HEALTH HISTORY AND PHYSICAL EXAMINATION

page 4

**SUBJECTIVE DATA**

☑ Information from patient
☐ Information from significant other

**OBJECTIVE DATA**

**MOVING**

☐ Seizures
☐ Dizziness
☐ Paralysis
☑ Sleep difficulty
☐ Sleepwalking

**Limits**
☐ Walking
☐ Bathing
☐ Recreational activities _____

Comments: *States she falls asleep easily but wakes after a "couple of hours" and can't fall asleep again.*

**Joint mobility**
☐ Moves all limbs
☑ Stiffness
☐ Equal grip
☐ Contractures
☐ Deformities
☐ Amputation

**Gait**
☑ Steady
☐ Unsteady
☐ Uses cane
☐ Uses walker
☐ Other: _____

Comments: _____

**RELATING AND CHOOSING**

☑ Married
☐ Separated
☐ Divorced
☐ Widowed
☐ Single

Most supportive relatives or friends *Husband*

☑ Alcohol use *rare*
How much *8 oz wine*
How often *about 1x/month*
☐ Substance abuse _____
Type _____
How much _____
How often _____

Observed behavior *Anxious and agitated*
Describe ability to comply with therapy (diet, medications, and so on) for chronic health problems (if applicable). *N/A*
_____
_____

**PERCEIVING AND COMMUNICATING**

☑ Hearing impairment
☑ Visual impairment

Comments: *Wears hearing aid and corrective lenses.*

Describe pupils. _____
☐ Blind _____
☐ Drainage from eyes *PERRLA*
☐ Drainage from ears _____
**Speech**
☑ Normal
☐ Slurred
☐ Aphasic
☐ Language barrier
Comments: _____

**LOC**
☑ Alert
☐ Lethargic
☐ Semiconscious
☐ Unconscious

# Functional health care patterns

This list shows you all the functional health care patterns along with the areas you need to assess for each.

**Cognition and perception**
☐ Mental status
☐ Vision
☐ Hearing
☐ Speech
☐ Pain

**Health perception and management**
☐ Chief complaint
☐ Medical history
☐ Allergies
☐ Medication use
☐ Use of community resources

**Role and relationships**
☐ Occupation
☐ Employment status
☐ Support systems

**Nutrition and metabolism**
☐ Diet
☐ Appetite
☐ Fluid intake
☐ Condition of teeth
☐ Use of dentures
☐ Eating disorders
☐ Skin, healing problems

**Elimination**
☐ Bowel habits
☐ Bladder habits
☐ Incontinence
☐ Use of assistive devices

**Activity and exercise**
☐ Self-care capabilities
☐ Activity tolerance
☐ Use of assistive devices

**Sleep and rest**
☐ Sleep habits
☐ Sedative use

**Sexuality and reproduction**
☐ Self-examination of breasts or testes
☐ Menses
☐ Sexual concerns

**Coping and stress tolerance**
☐ Major concerns
☐ Past coping strategies

**Values and beliefs**
☐ Cultural practices
☐ Religion

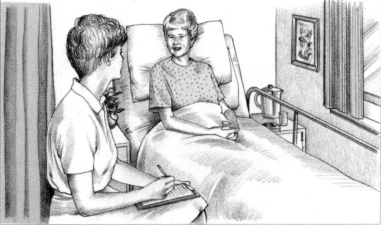

CHARTING

## Documenting functional health care patterns

Below you'll see one page of an assessment form that's organized by functional health care patterns. The sequence of health care patterns varies among forms.

### COGNITION AND PERCEPTION                                    page 2

**Mental status**
- ☑ Alert and oriented
- ☐ Lethargic
- ☐ Depressed
- ☐ Unresponsive
- ☐ Aphasic
- ☐ Combative

Confused
- ☐ Periodically
- ☐ At night
- ☐ At all times

**Vision**
- ☐ Normal
- ☐ Left impaired
- ☐ Right impaired
- ☑ Eyeglasses
- ☐ Contacts
- ☐ Prosthesis
- ☐ Left cataract
- ☐ Right cataract
- ☐ Glaucoma
- ☐ Left blind
- ☐ Right blind

**Hearing**
- ☐ Normal
- ☐ Hearing aid
- ☐ Left impaired
- ☑ Right impaired
- ☐ Left deaf
- ☐ Right deaf
- ☐ Tinnitus

**Speech**
- ☑ Normal
- ☐ Slurred
- ☐ Garbled
- ☐ Expressive aphasia
- ☐ Language barrier
- Language spoken _English_

**Pain**
- ☑ None
- ☐ Acute
- ☐ Chronic
- Describe pain and its management. _____

### COPING AND STRESS TOLERANCE

Describe patient's concerns about hospitalization.
_Anxious about possible diagnosis._
Identify coping methods used previously.
_Relies on husband for support._
Describe any major loss or change in the last year.
_Moved to area 6 months ago._

### VALUES AND BELIEFS

☐ Cultural practices _____
**Religion**
- ☐ Catholic
- ☑ Protestant
- ☐ Jewish
- ☐ None
- ☐ Other _____
Religious restrictions _None_
- ☐ Clergy visit requested
- ☐ Organ donation information

### ROLE AND RELATIONSHIPS

Occupation _Homemaker_
**Employment status**
- ☐ Employed
- ☐ Unemployed
- ☐ Short-term disability
- ☐ Long-term disability
- ☐ Retired

**Support systems**
- ☑ Spouse or family members
- ☐ Family at same residence
- ☐ Neighbors or friends
- ☐ Other _____
Describe concerns the family has about hospitalization. _____

CHARTING

## Documenting discharge planning

How and where you document your discharge planning will depend on the policy at the health care facility where you work. Here's one of the more common ways of documenting this information—using a designated section of an initial assessment form (usually the last page).

---

### DISCHARGE PLANNING NEEDS

Occupation _Homemaker_      Language spoken _English_

Patient lives with _Husband_

Self-care capabilities _Needs assistance_

**Assistance available**
☑ Cooking      ☑ Cleaning      ☑ Shopping

☐ Dressing changes/treatments _N/A_

**Medication administration routes**
☑ P.O.      ☐ I.M.      ☐ Other: _____
☐ I.V.      ☐ S.C.

**Dwelling**
☐ Apartment      ☑ Inside steps (number) _14_      ☑ Bathrooms (number) _2_ (location) _lower floor (off bedroom)_
☑ Private home
☐ Single room
☐ Institution      ☑ Kitchen gas stove      ☑ Telephones (number) _4_ (location) _den, living room, bedroom, kitchen_
☐ Elevator      (electric stove)
☑ Outside steps (number) _4_      wood stove other

**Transportation**
☑ Drives own car      ☐ Takes public transportation      ☐ Relies on family member or friend

**After discharge, patient will be:**
☐ Home alone      ☑ Home with family      ☐ Other: _____

**Patient has had help from:**
☐ Visiting nurse      ☐ Housekeeper      ☑ Other: _Husband_
Anticipated needs _Will need help with household chores._

Social service requests _for household help_
Date contacted _12/1/91_

When this occurs, base your initial assessment on your observations and physical examination of the patient. When documenting your findings, be sure to write something such as "Unable to obtain complete data at this time." Otherwise, it might appear that you failed to perform a complete assessment.

Try to obtain missing information as soon as possible, when the patient's condition improves or family members or other secondary sources are available. Be sure to record how and when you obtained the missing data. Depending on your facility's policy, you may record the information on the progress notes, or you may return to the initial assessment form and add the new information along with the date and your signature. Both methods have advantages and disadvantages.

Adding to the initial assessment form makes it easy to retrieve the data when it's needed — either during the patient's hospitalization or after discharge for quality assurance. Putting the information into the nursing progress notes aids in the day-to-day communication with others who read the notes but makes it difficult to retrieve the data later.

Remember, when you add information to complete an initial assessment, be sure to revise your nursing care plan accordingly.

# Ongoing assessment

Your assessment of a patient, of course, is a continuous process. Reassessment lets you evaluate the effectiveness of your nursing interventions and determine your patient's progress toward the desired outcomes. Effective documentation of your assessment findings facilitates communication with other health care practitioners, allowing you to plan the most appropriate patient care.

How often should you reassess a patient? That depends primarily on his condition. However, the JCAHO has a list of suggestions you can use as a basis for reassessing certain types of patients. (See *When to reassess,* page 84.) Your health care facility's policy should also define specific conditions under which you must reassess — for instance, when a patient is transferred to another unit.

**Planned reassessment**
A planned reassessment provides the routine data you must obtain to evaluate a patient on a daily basis. On a medical-surgical unit, this may include reviewing the patient's mental status, respiratory status, vital signs, skin integrity, self-care capabilities, appetite, and fluid balance as well as psychosocial factors. You'll also need to regularly reassess environmental factors and his learning and discharge needs. Based on the patient's condition, your nursing care plan may specify other reassessments as well.

At some facilities, health care team members must meet every 2 or 3 days during a patient's hospital stay to discuss and update discharge plans. At these meetings, staff representatives from various departments — including nursing, medicine, social service, physical therapy, and dietary — evaluate the patient's progress toward established goals and revise the care plan, as needed. Records of these meetings are maintained in the clinical record to ensure communication with other team members.

## When to reassess

The JCAHO suggests the following time intervals for patient reassessment. Keep in mind that these are minimum standards; some patients may need more frequent assessment.

| TYPE OF PATIENT | WHEN TO REASSESS |
| --- | --- |
| Patient with active GI bleeding | Continuously on a one-to-one basis |
| Suicidal patient | Continuously on a one-to-one basis |
| Patient with decreasing neurologic status | Every 15 minutes |
| Patient in labor | Every 15 minutes |
| Stable medical-surgical patient | Every 24 hours |
| Long-term care patient | Weekly |
| Patient in rehabilitation | Every 2 weeks |
| Same-day surgery patient | On return from recovery room and immediately before discharge |

### Unplanned reassessment

An unplanned reassessment occurs whenever the patient's condition or circumstances change unexpectedly. For example, suppose a patient with no previous cardiac dysfunction suddenly develops chest pain. You'd perform a complete assessment and schedule future cardiac reassessments according to the revised care plan. Or suppose you're caring for an elderly patient whose wife is his primary home caregiver. If his wife suddenly becomes incapacitated, you'd need to perform an unplanned reassessment of the patient's discharge needs to accommodate this change.

## Documenting ongoing assessment

You'll usually document ongoing assessment data on flow sheets or in narrative notes on the patient's progress report. Ideally, you should use flow sheets to document all routine assessment data and nursing interventions. That way, you can shorten the narrative notes to include only information regarding the patient's progress toward achieving desired outcomes, and any unplanned assessments.

Flow sheets come in many varieties, including temperature graphs and intake and output forms. When used to record routine assessment data, flow sheets can be a quick and consistent way to highlight trends in the patient's condition. A flow sheet for documenting information about a patient's skin integrity, for instance, will clearly show the progression of any pressure ulcers or reddened areas.

Because flow sheets are legally accepted components of the patient's clinical record, they must be documented correctly. Give yourself enough time to evaluate each piece of information on the flow sheet. And keep in mind that it must accurately reflect the patient's current clinical status. (See *Completing an assessment flow sheet,* pages 86 and 87.)

In some cases, you'll find that recording only the information requested on a flow sheet won't be sufficient to give a complete picture of the patient's status. When this occurs, record additional information in the space provided on the flow sheet. If additional information isn't necessary, draw a line through the space. Doing so indicates that, in your judgment, further information isn't required. If your flow sheet doesn't have additional space and you need to record more information, use the nurses' progress notes.

# Developing assessment forms

If you're developing a new assessment form or revising a current one, consider the following questions:
• What data from the health history and physical examination are currently included?
• Is this acceptable, or is more information needed to ensure quality?
• What problems exist with the current documentation system?
• What types of changes would help correct these problems?

## Development guidelines

If your health care facility uses a computerized documentation system, invite staff members involved in designing and programming the system to participate in discussions about changing it. To develop an effective assessment form, keep in mind the following guidelines:
• If your facility uses a specific nursing theory or framework for rendering nursing care, make sure the assessment form reflects it.
• If the current assessment form is modeled on a medical format, change it to reflect the nursing process. Organize the new assessment form according to human response patterns, functional health care patterns, or another nursing system.
• Ask staff members who will be using the form to evaluate the organizational formats and decide which they prefer. Invite them to share their ideas about how best to organize and document assessment data.

*(Text continues on page 88.)*

## Completing an assessment flow sheet

Most assessment flow sheets cover the categories of information shown below.

**ASSESSMENT FLOW SHEET**

Date  1/10/92

| DIET | | | |
|---|---|---|---|
| Meal | | Amount eaten | |
| Breakfast | | 100 % | |
| Lunch | | 90 % | |
| Dinner | | 90 % | |

☑ By himself
☐ With help
☐ With NG tube

| HYGIENE | 7-3 | 3-11 | 11-7 |
|---|---|---|---|
| By himself | SK | Jm | |
| With some help | | | |
| With complete help | | | |
| Shower | | | |
| Oral care | SK | Jm | |
| P.M. care | | Jm | |
| Catheter care | | | |

| ACTIVITY & REST | | | |
|---|---|---|---|
| On complete bed rest | | | |
| Turn q 2 hr | | | |
| OOB (chair) | | | |
| BRP | SK | Jm | BD |
| Walking | SK | Jm | BD |

| ELIMINATION | | | |
|---|---|---|---|
| Normal voiding | SK | Jm | BD |
| Has catheter | | | |
| Incontinent | | | |
| Bowel movement | | | |
| Emesis | | | |

| PULSE | | | |
|---|---|---|---|
| Regular | SK | Jm | BD |
| Irregular | | | |
| Strong | SK | Jm | BD |
| Weak | | | |

| MUSCULOSKELETAL | | | |
|---|---|---|---|
| Moves all limbs | SK | Jm | BD |
| Weak | | | |
| Paralyzed | | | |
| Paresthetic | | | |

| RESPIRATORY | 7-3 | 3-11 | 11-7 |
|---|---|---|---|
| Respirations | | | |
| Within normal limits | SK | Jm | BD |
| Shallow | | | |
| Deep | | | |
| Labored | | | |
| Respiratory rate | | | |
| Within normal limits | SK | Jm | BD |
| Slow | | | |
| Rapid | | | |
| Breath sounds | | | |
| Clear | SK | Jm | BD |
| Moist | | | |
| Wheezing | | | |
| Coughing | | | |

| SKIN | | | |
|---|---|---|---|
| Temperature | | | |
| Cool | | | |
| Warm | SK | Jm | BD |
| Hot | | | |
| Turgor | | | |
| Good | SK | Jm | BD |
| Fair | | | |
| Poor | | | |
| Edematous | | | |
| Moisture | | | |
| Dry | SK | Jm | BD |
| Moist | | | |
| Diaphoretic | | | |
| Color | | | |
| Within normal limits | SK | Jm | BD |
| Pale | | | |
| Ashen | | | |
| Cyanotic | | | |
| Flushed | | | |
| Jaundiced | | | |

| MENTAL STATUS | | | |
|---|---|---|---|
| Alert | SK | Jm | BD |
| Oriented × 3 | SK | Jm | BD |
| Disoriented | | | |
| Lethargic | | | |

## ASSESSMENT FLOW SHEET                                                    page 2

| BEHAVIOR | 7-3 | 3-11 | 11-7 |
|---|---|---|---|
| Cooperative | SK | Jm | BD |
| Uncooperative | | | |
| Anxious | | | |
| Withdrawn | | | |
| Combative | | | |
| Depressed | | | |
| **SPEECH** | | | |
| Clear | SK | Jm | BD |
| Slurred | | | |
| Rambling | | | |
| Aphasic | | | |
| Inappropriate | | | |
| **SLEEP** | | | |
| Sleeps well | | | BD |
| Sleeps intermittently | | | |
| Awake most of time | SK | Jm | |
| **GENERAL INFORMATION** | | | |
| In restraints | | | |
| Eggcrate-like mattress | | | |
| Side rails up | | | BD |
| In traction | | | |
| Under isolation precautions | | | |
| Above not applicable | SK | Jm | |

| WOUND | 7-3 | 3-11 | 11-7 |
|---|---|---|---|
| Type | | | |
| Size | | | |
| Appearance | | | |
| Sutures and drains | | | |
| Treatments | | | |
| Not applicable | SK | Jm | BD |
| **TUBES** | | | |
| Type | | | |
| Location | | | |
| Drainage | | | |
| Irrigation | | | |
| Not applicable | SK | Jm | BD |
| **I.V. THERAPY** | | | |
| I.V. site | (R)hand SK | (R)hand Jm | (R)hand BD |
| Catheter size | 20G. angio SK | 20G. angio Jm | 20G. angio BD |
| Tubing change | 10:00 a.m. SK | | |
| Site appearance | no redness or swelling SK | no redness or swelling Jm | no redness or swelling BD |
| Not applicable | | | |

| Signature and status | Initials |
|---|---|
| Sally Kendall, RN | SK |
| Janice Miller, RN | Jm |
| Brenda Draw, RN | BD |

• List all information the assessment form must include. Make sure you cover the six factors mandated by the JCAHO.

• Use a combination of documentation styles. Decide which style is most appropriate for each type of information included in the assessment form. For instance, you might use the *narrative note* to document the patient's chief complaint and his concerns about the impact of the hospitalization on himself and his family members. Generally, the *standardized open-ended style* works best when documenting health history information, such as medications, allergies, and psychosocial history. The *standardized close-ended style* works best for the review of body systems, biophysical data, and self-care capabilities.

• Include separate headings for listings of patient problems, nursing diagnoses, patient-teaching needs, discharge planning needs, and safety needs (such as potential for falling or suicide precautions).

• Have several staff members test the assessment form to make sure documentation can be completed easily.

• After you develop the assessment form, write procedure guidelines for using it. Provide clear explanations and completed examples for each section.

• Ask co-workers not involved in developing the assessment form to analyze both it and the guidelines. This helps identify potentially confusing sections that require more detailed explanation or revision.

## Suggested readings

Barnes, E. "When Will We Get It Right?....Care Plans Bear No Relation to the Assessment," *Nursing Times* 86(4):64, January 1990.

Carroll-Johnson, R.M., ed. *Classification of Nursing Diagnoses: Proceedings of the Eighth Conference North American Nursing Diagnosis Association.* Philadelphia: J.B. Lippincott Co., 1989.

Christensen, P.J., and Kenney, J.W. *Nursing Process Application of Conceptual Models.* St. Louis: C.V. Mosby Co., 1990.

Cline, A. "Streamlined Documentation Through Exceptional Charting," *Nursing Management* 20(2):62-64, February 1989.

Fox-Ungar, E., et al. "Documentation: Communicating Professionalism," *Nursing Management* 20(1):65-66, 68, 70, January 1989.

Jester, D.L. "Try This New Trauma Assessment Form," *Nursing88* 18(3):46-47, March 1988.

Johnson, M. "Perspectives on Costing Nursing," *Nursing Administration Quarterly* 14(1):65-71, Fall 1989.

Montemuro, M. "CORE Documentation: A Complete System for Charting Nursing Care," *Nursing Management* 19(8):28-32, August 1988.

Murray, R.B., and Zentner, J.P. *Nursing Assessment and Health Promotion Strategies Through the Lifespan,* 4th ed. Englewood Cliffs, N.J.: Appleton & Lange, 1989.

Werley, H.H., et al. "Status of the Nursing Minimum Data Set and Its Relationship to Nursing Diagnosis, in *Classification of Nursing Diagnoses: Proceedings of the Eighth Conference.* Edited by Carroll-Johnson, R.M. Philadelphia: J.B. Lippincott Co., 1989.

# 5

# NURSING DIAGNOSES AND CARE PLANS

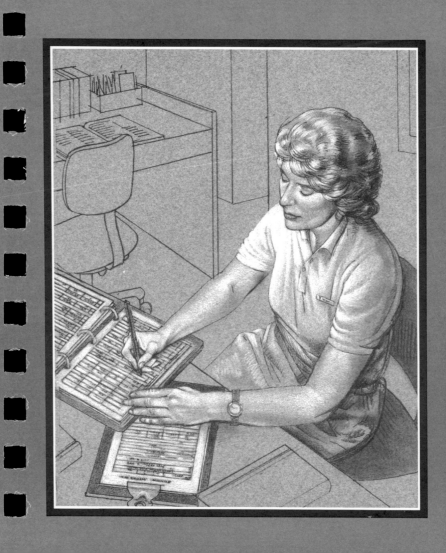

When you formulate nursing diagnoses and write a care plan for a patient, you're playing a key role in his recovery. To build a solid foundation for your care plan, you need to identify nursing diagnoses carefully. Then you must write a plan that not only fits your nursing diagnoses, but also fits your patient—taking into account his needs, age, developmental level, culture, strengths and weaknesses, and willingness and ability to take part in his care. Your plan should help him reach his highest functional level with minimal risk and without new problems. If he can't recover completely, your plan should help him cope physically and emotionally with his impaired or declining health. And, of course, you need to document all of this—carefully and completely.

That's a tall order. But this chapter will help you fill it by explaining the nursing diagnosis and planning processes and showing you how to document them most effectively. The first section covers how to formulate nursing diagnoses. Next comes a section on how to rank these diagnoses so you treat your patient's most urgent problems first. The third section reviews how to develop realistic expected outcomes—goals your patient should reach by or before discharge so he can function as effectively as possible. In the fourth section, you'll read about choosing the nursing interventions that will help your patient reach those expected outcomes. The next section explains how to write care plans. As you'll see, the discussion includes how to use protocols to make planning and documentation more efficient and how to document your patient teaching and discharge planning. The final section looks at case management, a comprehensive way of caring for a patient that attempts to meet both clinical and financial goals.

# Formulating nursing diagnoses

Unlike a medical diagnosis, which focuses on the patient's pathophysiology or illness, a nursing diagnosis focuses on the patient's responses to illness. (See *Nursing diagnoses: Avoiding the pitfalls.*)

## Types of nursing diagnoses

Depending on the policy of your health care facility, you'll either use standardized diagnoses or formulate your own diagnoses.

*Using standardized diagnoses.* In an effort to make nursing diagnoses consistent, several organizations have developed standardized lists, which are used by a growing number of health care facilities. The North American Nursing Diagnosis Association (NANDA) has developed the most widely accepted of these lists. NANDA categorizes nursing diagnoses according to the human response patterns of exchanging, communicating, relating, valuing, choosing, moving, perceiving, knowing, and feeling. NANDA meets every 2 years to consider new diagnoses.

Diagnoses can also be categorized according to nursing models, such as the one developed by Marjory Gordon. In this model, nursing diagnoses correspond to functional health patterns. Other ways of categorizing diagnoses—for instance, according to Orem's universal self-care demands—may also be used. Or your health care facility or unit can establish its own list of nursing diagnoses, categorizing them according to medical diagnoses and surgical procedures, for example.

No accrediting organization requires the use of standardized diagnoses. But by using a nationally accepted list like the NANDA list, health care facilities help establish a common language for nursing diagnoses—making communication easier and diagnosing more precise.

***Formulating your own nursing diagnoses.*** Developing your own diagnoses takes more effort than using standardized ones. But some nurses prefer this approach because they find the standardized diagnoses incomplete or their language overly formal or abstract. Such an approach can also help you characterize a problem that standardized diagnoses don't readily address.

### Deciding on a diagnosis

Before using or developing nursing diagnoses, you must evaluate relevant assessment data. You'll usually find this data on a standardized assessment form that groups related information into categories. Looking at the data in these groupings lets you determine which patient needs require nursing intervention. (See *Evaluating assessment data,* page 92.)

***Components of the diagnosis.*** Once you've examined the assessment data, you're ready to devise your nursing diagnoses. A diagnosis usually has three components: the human response or problem, related factors, and signs and symptoms.

*Human response or problem.* The first part of a diagnosis, the human

## Nursing diagnoses: Avoiding the pitfalls

To avoid common mistakes when formulating your nursing diagnoses, follow these guidelines:

☐ *Use nursing diagnoses, not medical diagnoses or interventions.* Terms such as angioplasty and coronary artery disease belong in a medical diagnosis—not in a nursing diagnosis.

☐ *Use all relevant assessment data.* If you just focus on the physical assessment, for instance, you might miss psychosocial or cultural information relevant to your diagnoses.

☐ *Take enough time to analyze the assessment data.* If you rush, you might easily miss something important.

☐ *Interpret the assessment data accurately.* Make sure you follow established norms, professional standards, and interdisciplinary expectations. Also, don't let your biases interfere with your interpretation of information. For instance, don't assume your patient is exaggerating if he states that he feels pain during what you would consider a painless procedure. If possible, have the patient verify your interpretation.

☐ *Keep data up-to-date.* Don't stop assessing and updating your diagnoses after the initial examination. As the patient's condition changes, so should your evaluation.

response, identifies an actual or potential problem that can be affected by nursing care. For instance, if assessment information on a patient with osteoarthritis shows that he has trouble moving, you might turn to the NANDA list, look under the human response pattern of moving, and identify the problem as impaired physical mobility. If the NANDA list doesn't provide a label that fits a patient's problem or if

**Evaluating assessment data**

To formulate your nursing diagnoses, you must evaluate the essential assessment information. These questions will help you quickly zero in on the appropriate data.

- Which signs and symptoms does the patient have?
- Which assessment findings are abnormal for this patient?
- How do particular behaviors affect the patient's well-being?
- What strengths or weaknesses does the patient have that affect his health status?
- Does he understand his illness and treatment?
- How does the patient's environment affect his health?
- Does he want to change his state of health?
- Do I need to gather any further information for my diagnoses?

your facility doesn't use standardized diagnoses, create your own label for the patient's condition.

*Related factors.* The second part of the nursing diagnosis identifies related factors. Such factors may precede, contribute to, or simply be associated with the human response. But no matter how they relate, these factors make your diagnosis more closely fit the particular patient and help you choose the most effective interventions.

For example, for your patient with osteoarthritis you may write "Impaired physical mobility related to pain and depression." For a patient with the same problem but a different related factor—a fractured tibia, for instance—you may write "Impaired physical mobility related to fractured tibia." Based on these re-

lated factors, you'd intervene differently for these two patients.

When you can't determine the related factors, write "related to unknown etiology" and modify your diagnosis as you obtain more information. To save charting time, use the standard abbreviation R/T for "related to" when writing your nursing diagnoses.

*Signs and symptoms.* Finally, a complete nursing diagnosis includes the signs and symptoms—or defining characteristics, as NANDA calls them—that led you to the diagnosis. You'll draw these from the assessment data. Not all nurses include signs and symptoms in their diagnoses but, like related factors, they help tailor the nursing diagnosis to the particular patient.

To help keep the nursing diagnosis brief, choose only the key characteristics. You can list them after the human response and related factors. For instance, you might write "Impaired thought processes R/T uncompensated perceptual cognitive impairment. Defining characteristics: short attention span during conversation; minimal speech; confused, oriented to person."

Alternatively, you can join the signs and symptoms to the first part of the nursing diagnosis with the words "as evidenced by," abbreviated AEB. For example, you'd write "Fluid volume excess R/T increased sodium intake AEB edema, weight gain, shortness of breath, and $S_3$ heart sounds."

## Setting priorities

Once you've made your nursing diagnoses, you'll need to rank them based on which problems require more immediate attention. Whenever possible, you should include the patient in this process. Maslow's hierarchy of needs is generally accepted as the basis for setting priorities. (See *Maslow's hierarchy of needs,* page 94.)

Typically, the first nursing diagnosis will stem from the primary medical diagnosis or from the patient's chief complaint. This nursing diagnosis points out a threat to the patient's physical well-being — sometimes to his life. For a patient who has a primary medical diagnosis of congestive heart failure (CHF), for instance, you'd give the first priority to the nursing diagnosis of decreased cardiac output R/T decreased contractility and altered heart rhythm.

Related nursing diagnoses come

next. These define problems that pose less immediate threats to the patient's well-being. For instance, you may have also selected for the CHF patient the nursing diagnosis of fluid volume excess R/T compromised regulatory mechanism.

Then, you'll usually list nursing diagnoses that refer to the patient's psychosocial, emotional, or spiritual needs. For the CHF patient, a nursing diagnosis of anxiety R/T possible loss of employment doesn't carry the same urgency as the previous two nursing diagnoses.

But just because a nursing diagnosis has a lower priority doesn't mean that you should wait to intervene until you've resolved all the higher priority problems. By helping the CHF patient cope with anxieties about losing his job, for example, you may speed his recovery — helping to resolve problems related to his physical well-being.

## Developing expected outcomes

After you've established and ranked nursing diagnoses, you're ready to develop expected outcomes, an increasingly important planning step. Based on nursing diagnoses, expected outcomes are goals the patient should reach as a result of planned nursing interventions. (Once achieved, an expected outcome is called a patient outcome.) You may find that one nursing diagnosis requires more than one expected outcome.

An outcome can specify an improvement in the patient's ability to function — an increase in the distance he can walk, for example. Or

## Maslow's hierarchy of needs

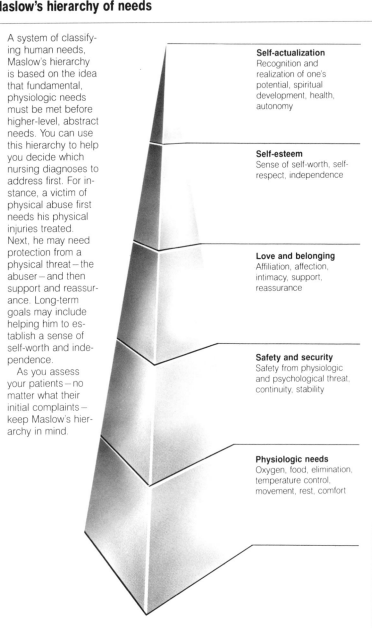

A system of classifying human needs, Maslow's hierarchy is based on the idea that fundamental, physiologic needs must be met before higher-level, abstract needs. You can use this hierarchy to help you decide which nursing diagnoses to address first. For instance, a victim of physical abuse first needs his physical injuries treated. Next, he may need protection from a physical threat — the abuser — and then support and reassurance. Long-term goals may include helping him to establish a sense of self-worth and independence.

As you assess your patients — no matter what their initial complaints — keep Maslow's hierarchy in mind.

**Self-actualization**
Recognition and realization of one's potential, spiritual development, health, autonomy

**Self-esteem**
Sense of self-worth, self-respect, independence

**Love and belonging**
Affiliation, affection, intimacy, support, reassurance

**Safety and security**
Safety from physiologic and psychological threat, continuity, stability

**Physiologic needs**
Oxygen, food, elimination, temperature control, movement, rest, comfort

## Writing an outcome statement

An outcome statement should consist of four components:

| B | M | C | T |
|---|---|---|---|
| **Behavior:** a desired behavior for the patient. This behavior must be observable. | **Measure:** criteria for measuring the behavior. The criteria should specify how much, how long, how far, and so on. | **Condition:** the conditions under which the behavior should occur. | **Time:** the time by which the behavior should occur. |

As indicated, the two outcome statements below have these four components.

| Ambulate | 25 feet | with walker | by 1/6/92 |
|---|---|---|---|

| Drink | 300 ml of water, | unassisted, | by noon, 1/9/92 |
|---|---|---|---|

an outcome can specify an amelioration of a problem, such as a reduction of pain. Each outcome should call for the maximum realistic improvement for a particular patient.

### Writing outcome statements

Ideally, an outcome statement should include four components: the specific behavior that will demonstrate the patient has reached his goal, criteria for measuring the behavior, the conditions under which the behavior should occur, and the time by which the behavior should occur. (See *Writing an outcome statement.*)

When you're writing outcome statements, follow these guidelines: Make your statements specific, focus on the patient, let the patient help you, take medical orders into ac-

count, adapt the outcome to the circumstances, and change your statements as necessary.

***Make your statements specific.*** If someone writes a statement such as "Understand relaxation techniques," you don't have much to go on. How do you observe a patient's understanding? A more specific statement such as "Practice progressive muscle relaxation techniques unassisted for 15 minutes daily by 12/10/91" tells you exactly what to look for when assessing the patient's progress. (Also see *Writing outcomes more efficiently,* page 96.)

***Focus on the patient.*** Make sure the outcome statement reflects the patient's behavior — not your intervention. The statements "Medication

## Writing outcomes more efficiently

Save yourself charting time by including only the essentials in your outcome statements. For instance, you don't need to refer to the patient, as this statement does: "Patient will demonstrate insulin self-administration, unassisted, by 12/15/91." You can simply drop the first two words of the statement — the reader knows you're referring to the patient. You only need to specify if you're referring to someone else.

Also, use accepted abbreviations wherever possible. For instance, if your health care facility uses relative dates, use abbreviations like HD2 for hospital day 2 or POD3 for postoperative day 3.

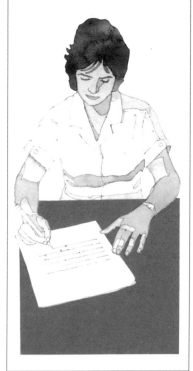

brings chest pain relief" and "Nurse to change patient position every 2 hours to promote comfort" don't say anything about the patient's behavior. A proper statement would be "Express relief of chest pain within 1 hour of receiving medication."

*Let the patient help you.* If the patient has a part in developing outcome statements, he's more motivated to achieve his goals. And his input — and the input of family members — can help you set realistic goals.

*Take medical orders into account.* Make sure you don't write outcome statements that ignore or contradict medical orders. For example, before writing the outcome statement "Ambulate 10 feet unassisted twice a day by 12/5/91," you should make sure the medical orders don't call for more restricted activity.

*Adapt the outcome to the circumstances.* Take into account the patient's coping ability, age, educational level, cultural influences, family support, living conditions, and socioeconomic situation. Also consider his anticipated length of stay when you're deciding on time limits for achieving goals. In some cases, you'll need to consider the health care setting itself. For instance, an outcome statement such as "Ambulate outdoors with assistance for 20 minutes t.i.d. by 12/14/91" may be unrealistic in a large city hospital.

*Change your statements as necessary.* Sometimes, you may need to revise even the most carefully written outcome statements. You may have to choose a later target date if the patient has trouble reaching his goal, for instance. Or you may need to change the goal to one the patient can reach more easily.

# Selecting interventions

Now, you're ready to select interventions—nursing actions that you and your patient agree will help him reach the expected outcomes. Base these interventions on the second part of your nursing diagnosis, the related factors. With a nursing diagnosis of impaired physical mobility R/T arthritic morning stiffness, for example, you'd select interventions that reduce or eliminate the patient's stiffness, such as mild stretching exercises. You'll need to write at least one intervention for each outcome statement.

## Considering potential interventions

You can come up with interventions in several ways. Start by considering ones that your patient or you have successfully tried before. Say your patient is having trouble sleeping. He knows he sleeps better at home if he has a glass of warm milk at bedtime. That could work as an intervention for the expected outcome, "Sleep through the night without medication by 12/3/91."

You can also pick interventions from standardized care plans, talk with your colleagues about interventions they've used successfully, or check nursing journals that discuss interventions for standardized nursing diagnoses. If these methods don't yield anything useful, try brainstorming.

## Guidelines for writing interventions

When you write your interventions,

be sure to follow these guidelines: Clearly state the action to be taken, make the intervention fit the patient, keep the patient's safety in mind, follow the rules of your health care facility, take other health care activities into account, and include the available resources.

*Clearly state the necessary action.* To ensure continuity of care, write your interventions with as much specific detail as possible. Note how and when to perform the intervention, and include any special instructions. An intervention such as "Promote comfort" doesn't tell another nurse what specific actions she should take. But "Administer ordered analgesic ½ hour before dressing change" lets her know exactly what to do and when to do it.

*Make the intervention fit the patient.* Keep in mind the patient's age, condition, developmental level, environment, and value system. For instance, if your patient is a vegetarian, you shouldn't write an intervention that requires him to eat lean meat to gain extra protein for healing. Instead, your intervention can call for him to eat legumes and dairy products.

*Keep the patient's safety in mind.* This means taking into account both the patient's physical and mental limitations. For instance, before teaching a patient to give himself a medication, make sure he's physically able to do so and that he can remember and follow the medication regimen.

*Follow the rules of your health care facility.* If your facility has a rule . that only nurses may administer medications, you obviously wouldn't write an intervention calling for the patient to administer hemorrhoidal suppositories as needed.

***Take other health care activities into account.*** Sometimes, other necessary activities may interfere with interventions you want to use. For example, you may want your patient to get plenty of rest on a day he has several diagnostic tests scheduled. In this case, you'd need to adjust your intervention.

***Include the available resources.*** If your patient needs to learn about his cardiac problem, use your health care facility's education department, literature from the American Heart Association, local support groups — anything that might help you carry out the intervention effectively. Then write the intervention to reflect the use of these resources.

# Writing your care plan

To document your nursing diagnoses, expected outcomes, and interventions, you can use either a traditional or a standardized care plan. You also may decide to use protocols along with one of these plans. In some cases, you can use protocols alone to demonstrate planned care. Your plan of care will also include your patient-teaching and discharge plans.

## Types of nursing care plans
Two basic types of care plans exist: traditional and standardized. No matter which you use, your plan should cover all nursing care from admission to discharge and should be a permanent part of the patient's clinical record. Be sure to write the care plan and put it into action as

soon as possible after the initial assessment. Then you can revise and update it throughout the patient's hospitalization. (See *Comparing care plans.*)

***Traditional care plan.*** Also called the individually developed care plan, the traditional care plan is written from scratch for each patient. After analyzing the assessment data, you'll either write the plan or enter it into a computer.

The basic form can vary, depending on the needs of the health care facility or department. Most forms have three main columns: one for nursing diagnoses, another for expected outcomes, and a third for interventions. Other columns allow you to enter the date you initiated the care plan, the target dates for expected outcomes, and the dates for review, revisions, and resolution. Most forms also have a place for you to sign or initial when you make an entry or a revision. Some forms still have columns for patient problems instead of nursing diagnoses, goals instead of expected outcomes, and nursing approaches or orders instead of interventions.

What you must include on these forms also varies. With shorter stays brought on by the advent of diagnosis-related groups (DRGs), most facilities require you to write only short-term outcomes that the patient should reach by or before discharge. But some facilities — particularly long-term care facilities — also want you to include long-term outcomes that reflect the maximum functional level the patient can reach. Such facilities frequently use forms that provide separate columns for the two types of outcomes. If they don't, you can label outcomes ''S'' for short-term and ''L'' for long-term. (See *Using a traditional care*

## Comparing care plans

The chart below highlights the advantages and disadvantages of the two basic types of nursing care plans.

| TYPE | ADVANTAGES | DISADVANTAGES |
|---|---|---|
| Traditional care plan | • Encourages fitting the care plan to the patient<br>• Can be easily adapted to fit the needs of the health care facility | • Can be time-consuming to write<br>• Can be time-consuming to update because whole plan must be rewritten<br>• May not be as comprehensive as a standardized care plan |
| Standardized care plan | • Saves writing time<br>• Provides carefully developed, efficient options for care<br>• Helps ensure that standards are met for quality assurance programs<br>• Can serve as a teaching tool for new graduates and nurses inexperienced in caring for a particular type of patient | • May not work well for a patient with more than one diagnosis; combining plans for such a patient may result in an excessively long plan<br>• Increases the risk that the care plan won't be tailored to the patient |

*plan,* page 100.)

***Standardized care plan.*** Developed to save documentation time and improve the quality of care, standardized care plans provide a series of interventions for patients with similar diagnoses. Most standardized care plans also supply root outcome statements. Some of these plans are classified by medical diagnoses or DRG; others, by nursing diagnoses.

The early versions of standardized care plans made no allowances for differences in patient needs. But current versions allow you to customize the plan to fit your patient's specific needs. In fact, they require you to explain how you've individualized the care plan. To use such a plan, you'll usually fill in the following information:

• related factors and signs and symptoms for a nursing diagnosis.

For instance, the form will provide a root diagnosis such as pain R/T. You might fill in "inflammation AEB grimacing, expressions of pain."
• the time limits for the outcomes. To a root statement of "Perform postural drainage without assistance," you might add "for 15 minutes immediately upon awakening in the morning by 12/11/91."
• frequency of interventions. You can complete an intervention such as "Perform passive range-of-motion exercises" with "twice a day: 1 × each in the morning and evening."
• specific instructions for interventions. For a standard intervention of "Elevate patient's head," you might specify "Before sleep, elevate the patient's head on three pillows."

When a patient has more than one diagnosis, the resulting combination of standardized care plans can be

*(Text continues on page 102.)*

## Using a traditional care plan

This sample shows how a traditional care plan organizes key information. Keep in mind that the care plans you'll use will have wider columns to allow more room for your notes.

| Date | Nursing diagnoses | Expected outcomes | Interventions | Revision (initials and date) | Resolution (initials and date) |
|------|-------------------|-------------------|---------------|------------------------------|--------------------------------|
| 12/3/91 | Decreased cardiac output R/T decreased contractility, fluid volume overload, and altered heart rhythm AEB dyspnea, crackles, and tachycardia. | Heart rate < 100 beats/min on auscultation by 12/4/91 | Monitor and document heart rate and rhythm, heart sounds, and BP. Note the presence or absence of peripheral pulses. Report any abnormalities. Administer cardiac medications as ordered and document pt.'s response. Observe for effectiveness and adverse reactions. | | |
| | | Lungs clear on auscultation by 12/5/91. | Ensure adequate oxygenation by placing pt. in semi-Fowler's position and administering supplemental O₂ as ordered. Monitor for signs and symptoms of hypoxemia, such as confusion, restlessness, dyspnea, arrhythmias, and cyanosis. MJ | | |

| Review dates | | Initials |
|--------------|-----------|----------|
| Date | Signature | MJ |
| 12/3/91 | Mary Johnson, RN | |

CHARTING

## Using a standardized care plan

The care plan below is for a patient with a nursing diagnosis of decreased cardiac output. To customize it to your patient, you'd complete the diagnosis—including signs and symptoms—and fill in the expected outcome. You'd also modify, add, or delete interventions as necessary.

Date
*12/3/91*

**Nursing diagnosis**
Decreased cardiac output R/T

*Decreased contractility, fluid volume overload, and altered heart rhythm AEB dyspnea, crackles, and tachycardia*

Target
date
*12/5/91*

**Expected outcome**
Adequate cardiac output AEB:
Heart rate _*< 100 beats/min*_
BP _*< 140/90 mm Hg*_
Pedal pulse _*palpable and regular*_
Radial pulse _*palpable and regular*_
Cardiac rhythm _*normal sinus*_
Cardiac index _*≤ 4.2 liters/min/m²*_
Pulmonary capillary wedge pressure (PCWP) _*≤ 12 mm Hg*_
Pulmonary artery pressure (PAP) _*≤ 20 mm Hg*_
SvO₂ _*≥ 60%*_
Urine output in ml/kg/hr _*≥ 0.3 ml/kg/hr*_

Date
*12/3/91*

**Interventions**
• Monitor ECG for rate and rhythm; note ectopic beats. If arrhythmias occur, note patient's response. Document and report findings and follow appropriate arrhythmia protocol.
• Monitor SvO₂, temperature, respirations, and central pressures (including PAP) continuously.
• Monitor other hemodynamic pressures (such as PCWP) q _*1*_ hr and p.r.n.
• Auscultate heart sounds and palpate peripheral pulses q _*4*_ hr and p.r.n.
• Monitor I & O q _*1*_ hr. Notify doctor if output < 30 ml/hr × 2 hr.
• Administer medications and fluids as ordered, noting effectiveness and adverse reactions. Titrate vasoactive drugs as needed. Follow appropriate vasoactive drug protocol to wean patient as tolerated.
• Monitor O₂ therapy or other ventilatory assistance.
• Decrease patient's activity to reduce O₂ demands. Increase as tolerated.
• Assess and document LOC. Assess for changes q _*1*_ hr and p.r.n.
• Additional interventions _*Inspect for pedal and sacral edema q 4 hr.*_

long and cumbersome. But computerized documentation can help. With computerized plans, you can pull only what you need from each one and combine them to make one manageable plan. Some computer programs simply provide a checklist of interventions you can use to build your own plan.

Keep in mind that standardized plans usually include only essential information. But most provide space for you to add further nursing diagnoses, expected outcomes, and interventions. (See *Using a standardized care plan,* page 101.)

## Protocols

A newer documentation tool, protocols give specific sequential instructions for treating patients with particular problems. Originally developed to help nurses manage equipment and provide specific treatments, protocols now are also used to manage patients with specific nursing diagnoses. (See *Using a protocol.*)

Protocols offer several advantages. Because they spell out the steps to follow for a patient with a particular nursing diagnosis, protocols can help you provide thorough care and ensure that the patient receives consistent care from all caregivers. More detailed protocols even specify what to teach the patient and what to document and include a reference section that lets you quickly determine how up-to-date they are. Some protocols also spell out the role of other health care professionals, helping all team members coordinate their efforts. And by supplying such comprehensive instruction, protocols help teach inexperienced staff members. Used in conjunction with other care plans or alone, protocols can also save documentation time.

*Using protocols.* Before you use a protocol, make sure you have the current version. If you give care according to an outdated version, you may be liable for not following your facility's policies and procedures. If you can't get a copy of the latest version, find out what changes have been made and update the version you have.

Use the protocols that best fit your patient. You'll use some protocols, such as the generic one for pain, for several patients. You'll use others rarely. For example, the protocol — Potential for violence: self-directed — applies mainly to patients in psychiatric settings. If you find that a protocol doesn't exist for a patient problem, you can help develop a new one. (See *Developing a protocol,* pages 106 and 107.)

Once you've selected a protocol, make sure you tailor it to fit your patient's needs. Cross out steps that don't apply to your patient and modify or add material as needed.

*Documenting protocols.* To document a protocol on a care plan, note in the interventions section that you'll follow the protocol. Write, for instance, "Follow impaired gas exchange protocol." Or list the protocols you plan to use on a flow sheet.

After you intervene, simply write in your progress notes that you followed the protocol, or check the protocol off on your flow sheet and initial it. The protocol itself usually remains at the nurses' station, but you should include a copy in the patient's record — especially if you've made changes to it.

## Patient-teaching plan

You'll also need to include a patient-teaching plan as part of your plan of care. You may either include this on

*(Text continues on page 107.)*

CHARTING

## Using a protocol

As this sample shows, a protocol gives specific instructions for providing thorough, consistent care.

---

### PATIENT CARE PROTOCOL

**Title:** Potential for altered nutrition: less than body requirements; Potential fluid volume deficit

**Personnel**
1. Assessment: RN
2. Planning: RN
3. Intervention: RN, LPN, nursing assistant
4. Patient teaching: RN, LPN, dietitian
5. Evaluation: RN
6. Complications: RN, LPN, nursing assistant, dietitian
7. Documentation: RN

**Competencies**
Caregiver must:
• be able to identify patients at risk for nutrition and fluid volume deficit
• be able to assess patients at risk for nutrition and fluid volume deficit
• have a basic understanding of these problems and their treatments
• be qualified to perform necessary interventions.

**Expected outcomes**
Patient will:
1. have decreased nausea, vomiting, or diarrhea.
2. take in adequate calories.
3. take in sufficient fluids.
4. demonstrate knowledge of his nutritional needs.
5. show these signs of adequate hydration: improved skin turgor, moist mucous membranes, increased urine output.
6. show these signs of adequate caloric intake: improved appetite, weight gain, increased energy.

**Supportive data**
1. Risk factors:
• hyperthermia, anorexia, nausea and vomiting, and diarrhea
• infectious or inflammatory processes
2. Signs and symptoms of nutrition and fluid volume deficit:
• dry mucous membranes
• poor skin turgor
• lethargy
3. Procedures for monitoring patients at risk for nutrition and fluid volume deficit include:
• measuring intake and output and weighing patient. I.V. equipment, total parenteral nutrition equipment, and scale may be used.
• performing a neurologic assessment to provide early clues to fluid volume deficit.

## Using a protocol (continued)

| Areas of responsibility | Nursing actions |
| --- | --- |
| 1. Assessment | 1.1 Assess general physical condition every 8 hours.<br>1.2 Assess neurologic status every 8 hours. Especially note subtle changes in behavior or LOC.<br>1.3 Assess daily caloric and fluid intake, using these guidelines:<br>• Good: Intake provides 50% or more of needed calories and fluids.<br>• Fair: Intake provides more than 20% and less than 50% of needed calories and fluids.<br>• Poor: Intake provides less than 20% of needed calories and fluids.<br>• None: Unable or refuses to eat or drink. |
| 2. Planning | 2.1 Collaborate with doctor to decide when to perform interventions that will help patient meet daily nutrition and fluid needs. Meet with dietitian to ensure reinforcement of nutritional counseling in preparation for discharge. |
| 3. Interventions | 3.1 Monitor intake, output, and weight.<br>3.2 Monitor bowel function.<br>3.3 Monitor results of laboratory studies (serum albumin, total protein, urine protein, glucose, acetone, nitrogen).<br>3.4 Observe patient and help him choose amount and types of foods and liquids.<br>3.5 Provide smaller but more frequent meals.<br>3.6 Help patient to a comfortable position at mealtimes.<br>3.7 Help patient with meals; feed patient if necessary.<br>3.8 Arrange for dietitian to assess patient's caloric requirements.<br>3.9 Offer fluids every 4 hours between meals; try to ensure a total daily intake of 3,000 ml unless contraindicated.<br>3.10 Provide parenteral fluids as ordered.<br>3.11 Provide nutritional supplements. |
| 4. Patient teaching | 4.1 Explain the need to take in sufficient calories to maintain adequate nutrition and the need to maintain adequate fluid balance.<br>4.2 Instruct the patient and family members about the patient's specific nutritional needs. |
| 5. Evaluation | 5.1 Evaluate nutritional and fluid status of patient every 8 hours and anytime a significant change in patient status or regimen occurs. |

CHARTING

## Using a protocol *(continued)*

| Areas of responsibility | Nursing actions |
|---|---|
| 6. Complications | 6.1 Observe for complications including:<br>• dehydration<br>• anemia<br>• malnutrition<br>• sepsis.<br>6.2 Notify doctor, document appropriately, continue assessment and interventions, and carry out additional doctor's orders. |
| 7. Documentation | 7.1 Document the following:<br>• Ongoing nutritional and fluid assessment data on nurses' progress sheet<br>• Nutritional and fluid status of patient on nurses' progress sheet<br>• Intake and output every 8 hours<br>• Vital signs as ordered by doctor but at least every 8 hours<br>• Patient teaching on nutritional and fluid needs<br>• Any complications and actions taken to correct them<br>• Daily weights on graphic record<br>• Type and amount of nutritional therapy on patient care flow sheet<br>• Type and amount of fluid therapy on I.V. therapy sheet every 8 hours and at completion of infusion. |

**Author(s):** Maria Rodriguez, RN

**References**
Bodinsky, G. "Fluid and Electrolyte Balance and the Patient with a Digestive Disorder," *Gastroenterology Nursing* 12(3):212-14, Winter 1990.
Brunner, L.S., and Suddarth, D.S. *Textbook of Medical-Surgical Nursing,* 6th ed. Philadelphia: J.B. Lippincott Co., 1988.
Buelow, J.M., and Jamieson, D. "Potential for Altered Nutritional Status in the Stroke Patient," *Rehabilitation Nursing* 15(5):260-63, September/October 1990.
Cox, H.C., et al. *Clinical Applications of Nursing Diagnosis.* Baltimore: Williams & Wilkins, 1989.
Holloway, N.M. *Medical-Surgical Care Plans.* Springhouse, Pa.: Springhouse Corp., 1988.
*Metabolic Problems.* NurseReview series. Springhouse, Pa.: Springhouse Corporation, 1988.
Sprauve, D. "Fluids, Electrolytes and Acid-base Balance," *Nursing90* 20(3):103, 105-07, March 1990.

**Distribution:** All patient care units
**Approval:** Alison Williams (Chairperson, Nursing Practice Council)
**Date:** 12/12/90
**Revision date:** 1/23/92

## Developing a protocol

When you need to develop a protocol, follow these guidelines for the various categories of information.

### Basic information

*Title:* Be specific. The title may be a nursing diagnosis or a description of the purpose of the protocol — for example, "Management of I.V. lidocaine drip."

*Personnel:* Specify who can perform each part of the protocol.

*Competencies:* State the knowledge and skills caregivers need to carry out the protocol.

*Expected outcomes:* List the specific outcomes you hope to achieve with the protocol.

*Supportive data:* Provide information needed to carry out the protocol, including key definitions, abbreviations used, specific equipment used, risk factors, and signs and symptoms. Also list accompanying procedures used to monitor or care for the patient.

### Areas of responsibility and nursing actions

The heart of the protocol, this section follows the nursing process. Each area of responsibility has corresponding nursing actions.

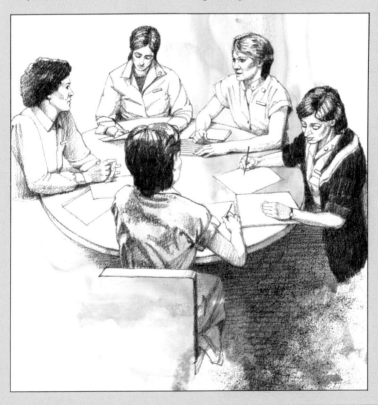

*1. Assessment:* Tell what to assess and how often to assess.
*2. Planning:* Explain planning that needs to be done by the nurse with other health care team members to meet daily patient needs and discharge planning needs.
*3. Interventions:* Include specific routine interventions and prevention measures.
*4. Patient teaching:* State exactly what the patient needs to be taught.
*5. Evaluation:* Explain what to evaluate and when to evaluate.
*6. Complications:* State complications that may develop and briefly explain how to manage them.
*7. Documentation:* State which information to include and when to document (at the beginning of each shift or every 2 hours, for example).

When writing nursing actions for these seven areas, follow these suggestions:
• Use action verbs, such as change, check, assess, stop, and notify.
• Write interventions in the order you'll perform them.
• Focus on nursing actions, not medical orders or policy statements.
• Make sure directives meet minimum standards to ensure safe, effective, appropriate care.

**Miscellaneous information**
*Author(s):* List all authors of the protocol.
*References:* Include written and other resources.
*Distribution:* Note whether the protocol is generic or applies to certain units, and specify those units.
*Approval:* Note who approved the protocol.
*Date:* Note the date of approval.
*Revision date:* Note the revision date.

your main plan or write a separate plan. Today, many health care facilities require a separate plan because of the emphasis placed on patient teaching by accrediting and regulatory organizations. The need to control costs and discharge patients earlier also calls for more extensive teaching plans.

***Purpose of the teaching plan.*** Besides identifying what the patient needs to learn and how he'll be taught, a teaching plan also sets criteria for evaluating how well he learns. The plan also helps all the patient's educators coordinate their teaching. Plus, it serves as legal proof that the patient received appropriate instruction and satisfies the requirements of regulatory agencies, such as the Joint Commission on Accreditation of Healthcare Organizations.

To make sure your teaching plan does all that it should, you must carefully organize what the patient needs to learn and how you'll provide the instruction and measure the results. Work closely with other health care team members as well as with the patient and his family to make the plan's content realistic and attainable during his stay. And include provisions for follow-up teaching at home.

Also, keep your patient-teaching plan flexible. Take into account such variables as the patient being unreceptive because of a poor night's sleep as well as your own daily time limits.

***Components of the plan.*** Although the scope of each teaching plan differs, all should contain the same elements:
• patient learning needs
• expected learning outcomes
• teaching content, organized from

the simplest concepts to the most complex
• teaching methods and tools.

*Patient learning needs.* Identifying learning needs helps you decide which outcomes you should establish for your patient. Be sure to take into account not only what you, the doctor, and other health care team members want the patient to learn, but also what he wants to learn.

*Expected learning outcomes.* As with your patient care outcomes, your expected learning outcomes should focus on the patient and be readily measurable.

Your patient's learning behaviors and the outcomes you develop fall into three categories:
• cognitive, relating to understanding
• psychomotor, covering manual skills
• affective, dealing with attitudes.

For a patient learning to give himself subcutaneous injections, identifying an injection site would be the cognitive outcome; giving the injection, the psychomotor outcome; and coping with the need for injections, the affective outcome. (See *Writing clear learning outcomes.*)

To help formulate precise, measurable outcomes, decide which evaluation techniques will best reveal the patient's progress. For cognitive learning, you might use questions and answers; for psychomotor learning, you might use return demonstration. To measure affective learning, which can be difficult because changes in attitudes develop slowly, you can use several evaluation techniques. To determine whether a patient has overcome his anxiety about giving himself an injection, you can ask him if he still feels anxious. You can also assess

## Writing clear learning outcomes

The patient's learning behaviors fall into three categories: cognitive, psychomotor, and affective. With these categories in mind, you can write clear, concise, expected learning outcomes. Remember, your outcomes should clarify what you're going to teach, indicate the behavior you expect to see, and set criteria for evaluating what the patient has learned.

Review the two sets of sample learning outcomes at the right for a patient with chronic renal failure. Notice that the outcomes in the well-phrased set start with a precise action verb, confine themselves to one task, and describe measurable and observable learning. In contrast, the poorly phrased goals may encompass many tasks and describe learning that's difficult or even impossible to measure.

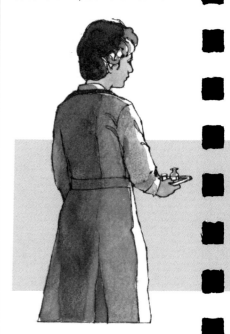

| WELL-PHRASED LEARNING OUTCOMES | POORLY PHRASED LEARNING OUTCOMES |
|---|---|

### Cognitive domain

The patient with chronic renal failure will be able to:

| | |
|---|---|
| • state when to take each prescribed drug. | • know his medication schedule. |
| • describe symptoms of elevated blood pressure. | • know when his blood pressure is elevated. |
| • list permitted and prohibited foods on his diet. | • realize his dietary restrictions. |

### Psychomotor domain

The patient with chronic renal failure will be able to:

| | |
|---|---|
| • take his blood pressure accurately, using a stethoscope and a sphygmomanometer. | • take his blood pressure. |
| • read a thermometer correctly. | • use a thermometer. |
| • collect a urine specimen, using sterile technique. | • bring in a urine specimen for laboratory studies. |

### Affective domain

The patient with chronic renal failure will be able to:

| | |
|---|---|
| • comply with dietary restrictions to maintain normal electrolyte values. | • appreciate the relationship of diet to renal failure. |
| • verbally express his feelings about adjustments to be made in the home environment. | • adjust successfully to limitations imposed by chronic renal failure. |
| • keep scheduled doctor appointments. | • realize the importance of seeing his doctor regularly. |

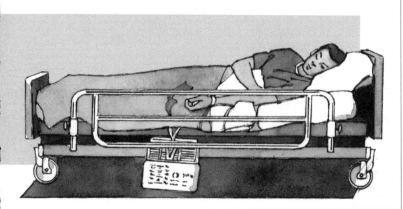

his willingness to perform the procedure. And you can observe whether he hesitates or shows other signs of stress while doing it.

*Teaching content.* Next, you'll need to select what to teach the patient to help him achieve the expected outcomes. As you make these decisions, be sure to include family members and other caregivers in your plan. Even if a patient will learn to care for himself, you can teach a family member how to provide physical and emotional support. You can also teach a family member to serve as a source of information in case the patient forgets some aspect of his care.

Once you've decided what to teach, carefully organize it. Start with the simplest concepts and work toward the more complex ones. You'll find this especially helpful for teaching a patient with little education or one who doesn't learn well by listening. (See *Tips for teaching patients.*)

*Teaching methods.* You'll also need to select the appropriate teaching method for your patient. You can probably plan to do most of your teaching on a one-to-one basis. This method gives you a chance to learn about your patient, build a relationship with him, and tailor your teaching to his learning needs.

But you can use other methods too—either in place of or in conjunction with one-on-one teaching. For instance, you may want to incorporate demonstration, practice, and return demonstration in your teaching plan. Role-playing can help involve your patient in learning, as can case studies, which call for him to evaluate how someone else with his disorder responds to different situations. Self-monitoring also involves

the patient because he must assess his situation and determine which aspects of his environment or behavior need correction. If you have several patients who need similar instruction, you can also try group teaching or lecturing. (For more information, see *Becoming a better teacher,* page 112.)

*Teaching tools.* Finally, you must include the teaching tools you intend to use. These tools—ranging from printed pamphlets to closed-circuit television programs—can help familiarize the patient with a topic.

When choosing your tools, focus on what will work best for the particular patient. For instance, if your patient likes to watch how something is done, he may respond best to a videotape of a procedure, a closed-circuit television demonstration, or a slide show. For a patient who prefers a hands-on approach, you might use a working model or let him handle the equipment he'll use. A computerized patient-teaching program may be best for a patient who likes to work interactively at his own pace. And some patients may simply want to read about their disorders.

Keep the abilities and limitations of your patient in mind as you choose. For instance, if you plan to provide him with written materials to reinforce your instructions, make sure he can understand them. (The average adult has only a seventh-grade reading level.)

To get the tools you need, consult the staff-development instructors on your unit, the health care facility's librarian, or staff specialists. If your facility doesn't have what you need, you might try the pharmaceutical and medical supply companies in your community. And don't overlook national associations and founda-

CHECKLIST

## Tips for teaching patients

To make your teaching as effective as possible, follow these suggestions:
☐ Use language that's appropriate for the patient's educational level or fluency in English. You're usually on safe ground if you select simple words with few syllables, keep your sentences short, and use action verbs.
☐ Express complex medical and scientific concepts in lay terms, and use analogies to make your meaning clear. Whenever possible, avoid complex clinical terms and abbreviations.
☐ Choose specific rather than general words when giving instructions. This is particularly important when giving directions for self-care, such as administering medications.
☐ Use examples and hypothetical cases to humanize your teaching.

☐ For clarity, break your information into large, distinct categories. You might say to the patient, "I have three important things to tell you today. Number one is . . . ."
☐ State your most important points first and last. Information given at the beginning and the end will be remembered best.
☐ Repeat important points. Don't be afraid to repeat them more than once if you suspect that the patient hasn't grasped them.
☐ To build confidence, help the patient reach his first learning outcome quickly. You can choose something simple, like taking his own pulse.
☐ Ask the patient if he understands what you've taught him. Evaluate both his verbal and nonverbal responses.

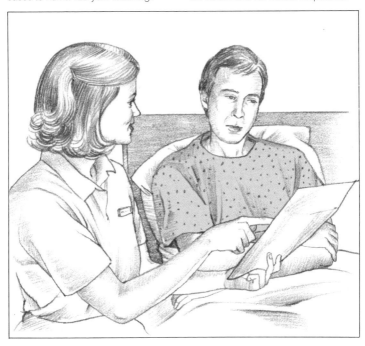

## Becoming a better teacher

These suggestions will help you improve your teaching skills.

□ Learn as much as you can about patient teaching by reading professional publications, attending staff-development and continuing education programs, and maintaining a broad range of professional contacts.

□ Ask the staff-development department to schedule classes that can benefit you and others on your unit.

□ If you're not up-to-date on a subject you must teach, ask the staff-development department to supply the names of specialists on the subject. Then call one for an appointment.

□ Observe more experienced nurses while they're teaching patients. What makes their teaching effective? What kind of rapport do they have with their patients? How do they reach difficult-to-teach patients? Which of their methods could you use effectively?

□ If you have a patient who's unusually difficult to teach, ask a colleague or a nursing consultant to do the teaching while you observe.

□ Ask a colleague whom you consider an especially good teacher to sit in while you teach. Afterward, ask her to offer pointers for your next teaching session. If you're uncomfortable having a third person present while you teach, try role-playing the session beforehand to smooth any rough edges in your presentation and help put you at ease for the actual session.

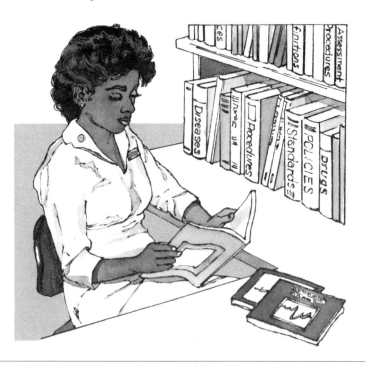

tions, such as the American Cancer Society. These organizations usually have large supplies of patient-education materials written with the layperson in mind.

***Documenting the patient-teaching plan.*** Several forms are available for documenting your patient-teaching plan. Many of them include the phases of the nursing process as they relate to patient education. (See *Using a patient-teaching flow sheet,* page 114.)

Patient-teaching plans come in two basic types. Like the traditional care plan, one type provides only the format and calls for you to come up with the plan. When a particular DRG requires extensive teaching, you may be able to use a standardized plan instead, checking off or dating steps as you complete them and adding or deleting information to individualize the plan.

Both types of plans include space for problems that may hinder learning, comments and evaluations, and dates and signatures. No matter which plan you use, it becomes a permanent part of the clinical record.

## Discharge planning

The final part of the planning process, the discharge plan has become more important in recent years because of the trend toward shorter hospital stays. You'll need to start your discharge planning the day your patient is admitted—or sooner for a planned admission. Such early planning can help avert problems.

***Responsibility for discharge planning.*** In some health care facilities, the social service department carries the major responsibility for discharge planning. Larger facilities may hire a discharge planner (possi-

bly a nurse) to take charge. But many facilities still require staff nurses to play the major role, sometimes along with continuing care coordinators.

Even if you don't have the primary responsibility for discharge planning, you still play an important part. You and other health care team members need to coordinate your efforts with the discharge planners or social service department. Typically, you'll do this at a multidisciplinary discharge conference, in which team members evaluate the patient's discharge needs, discuss appropriate plans, and evaluate his progress.

***Components of the plan.*** A discharge plan should note the anticipated length of stay and specify what the patient needs to learn, including:
• diet
• medications
• treatments
• physical activity limitations
• signs and symptoms to report to the doctor
• follow-up medical care
• equipment
• appropriate community resources and support groups.

As part of your plan, make sure the patient receives an instruction sheet to reinforce what he learns during patient teaching and what he needs to remember about follow-up care.

The discharge plan should also spell out future care, including the setting for it. Plus, the plan should note the patient's intended caregiver and support systems, actual or potential barriers to care, and any referrals.

***Documenting the discharge plan.*** How you document the discharge plan will depend on the policy at

CHARTING

## Using a patient-teaching flow sheet

Below you'll find the first page of a patient-teaching flow sheet. Such flow sheets let you quickly and easily tailor your teaching plan to fit your patient's needs.

**PATIENT-TEACHING FLOW SHEET**
**Diabetes mellitus**

**Problems affecting learning**
☐ None
☑ Fatigue or pain
☐ Communication problem

☐ Cognitive or sensory impairment
☐ Physical disability

☐ Lack of motivation
☐ Other _____
_____

**KEY**
**Learner**
P = patient
S = spouse
M = mother
F = father
D1 = daughter 1 _____
D2 = daughter 2 _____
S1 = son 1 _____
S2 = son 2 _____
O = other _____

**Teaching techniques**
D = demonstration
E = explanation
R = role-playing
**Teaching tools**
F = filmstrip
P = physical model
S = slide
V = videotape
W = written material

**Evaluation**
S = states understanding
D = demonstrates understanding
Dp = demonstrates understanding with physical coaching
Dv = demonstrates understanding with verbal coaching
T = passes written test
N = no indication of learning
NE = not evaluated

| LEARNING OUTCOMES | INITIAL TEACHING | | | | | | REINFORCEMENT | | | | | |
|---|---|---|---|---|---|---|---|---|---|---|---|---|
| | Date | Time | Learner | Techniques and tools | Evaluation | Initials | Date | Time | Learner | Techniques and tools | Evaluation | Initials |
| **Basic knowledge** | | | | | | | | | | | | |
| • Define diabetes mellitus (DM). | 1/9/92 | 10 a.m | P | E,W | S | JM | 1/11/92 | 11 a.m | P | E,W | S | JM |
| • List four symptoms of DM. | 1/9/92 | 10 a.m | P | E,W | S | JM | 1/11/92 | 11 a.m | P | E,W | S | JM |
| **Medication** | | | | | | | | | | | | |
| • State the action of insulin and its effects on the body. | 1/10/92 | 10 a.m. | P | E,W | S | JM | | | | | | |
| • List the three major classifications of insulin. Give their onsets, peaks, and durations. | 1/10/92 | 10 a.m | P | E,W,V | Dv | JM | | | | | | |
| • Demonstrate the ability to draw up insulin in a syringe and mix the correct amount. | | | | | | | | | | | | |

your health care facility. Some policies require you to include your assessment of discharge needs on the initial assessment form, then document the discharge plan itself on a separate form. At many facilities, you must include the discharge plan as a component of the discharge summary. Some forms used for discharge planning allow several members of the health care team to include information.

# Case management

A method of delivering health care that controls costs while still ensuring quality care, case management goes a step beyond planned care to managed care. It came into being after the government introduced the prospective payment system in 1983. Under this system Medicare pays the facility based on the patient's diagnosis—not on his length of stay or the number or types of services he receives. Thus, the facility loses money if it must pay more to treat the patient than Medicare says it should receive.

Such a system forces health care facilities to deliver cost-effective care—without compromising the quality of care. And the case management system proposes to help them do that by managing each patient's care to meet both clinical and financial goals.

**Your role in case management**
If you become a case manager, your role will expand beyond giving nursing care. You'll learn to manage a closely monitored and controlled system of multidisciplinary care. And you'll take on responsibility for outcomes, length of stay, and use of

resources throughout the patient's illness—not just during your shift.

**How the system works**
When a patient is assigned a particular DRG, he's also assigned a case manager. (In some facilities, a patient isn't assigned a DRG until after discharge—in which case, you'll need to make an educated guess about which DRG he'll be assigned.) Each DRG case management plan has standard outcome criteria and includes medical and nursing interventions as well as interventions from other disciplines.

As the case manager for a patient, you'll discuss the outcomes with the patient and his family, using the established time line for the patient's DRG. This time line should cover all the processes that must occur for the patient to reach the expected outcome, including tests, procedures, and patient teaching, and the resources such as social services the patient will need. If it doesn't, you'll adapt it as necessary to fit the patient's needs. If possible, you should do all this before the patient is even admitted, but you must complete these steps within the time limit set by your facility—usually 24 hours.

Once the patient is admitted, the multidisciplinary team evaluates his progress and suggests any necessary revisions, keeping in mind the need for continuity of care and the best use of resources. You'll document any variations in the time line, processes, or outcomes, along with the reasons for the changes. Plus, you'll keep a lookout for duplication of services and medical orders.

You must also start discharge planning, beginning an assessment of the patient's discharge needs at or before admission. And you're responsible for activating home health
(Text continues on page 118.)

## Following a critical path

The sample below shows you selected portions of a typical critical path, starting with the preoperative day on this page and then moving to the first two postoperative days on the next page.

---

### CRITICAL PATH

**Diagnosis:** Partial or total parotidectomy

**DRG length of stay:** 2.3 days

**Actual length of stay:** _____

**Expected outcomes**

By discharge, the patient will:
• state possible complications, troubleshooting measures, and appropriate resources.
• perform suture line care.
• explain measures for managing his pain.
• explain how to maintain his nutritional status.
• demonstrate eye care measures (if applicable).

| Nurse | Other health care providers | Patient and family |
|---|---|---|
| **Preoperative day** | | |
| • Performs assessment <br> • Explains case-management model and recovery pathway to patient <br> • Completes contract with patient and family <br> • Performs preoperative teaching <br> • Notifies social worker, if appropriate, and explains assessment and possible discharge needs to her | *Primary doctor* <br> • Performs physical examination <br> • Orders special studies, including blood work, ECG, chest X-rays <br> • Orders anesthesia clearance assessment <br><br> *Social worker* <br> • Consults with nurse (if appropriate) | *Patient and family* <br> • Sign contract <br> • Visit immediate postop care unit |

**CRITICAL PATH**                                                               page 3

| Nurse | Other health care providers | Patient and family |
| --- | --- | --- |

### Postoperative day (POD) 1

| Nurse | Other health care providers | Patient and family |
| --- | --- | --- |
| • Provides morning care while patient is on bed rest<br>• Sets up heparin lock on I.V. line<br>• Teaches suture line care<br>• Teaches eye care (if applicable)<br>• Encourages activity<br>• Monitors diet | *Primary doctor*<br>• Orders laboratory tests<br>• Orders advance in diet as tolerated<br>• Orders heparin lock on I.V. line<br>• Consults with ophthalmologist, radiation therapist, and dentist (as applicable)<br><br>*Ophthalmologist*<br>• Consults with doctor (if applicable)<br><br>*Radiation therapist*<br>• Consults with doctor (if applicable)<br><br>*Dentist*<br>• Consults with doctor (if applicable) | *Patient*<br>• Performs oral hygiene and incentive spirometry<br>• Demonstrates suture line care and eye care (if applicable)<br>• Ambulates q 4 hr p.r.n. |

### POD 2

| Nurse | Other health care providers | Patient and family |
| --- | --- | --- |
| • Continues to teach suture line care and eye care<br>• Continues to encourage activity and monitor diet. | *Dietitian*<br>• Performs nutrition assessment<br><br>*Speech pathologist*<br>• Performs nutrition assessment (if patient has difficulty swallowing) | *Patient*<br>• Performs morning self-care<br>• Continues to perform oral hygiene and incentive spirometry<br>• Demonstrates suture line care and eye care (if applicable)<br>• Ambulates q 4 hr p.r.n. |

care services — including obtaining personnel and equipment — well before discharge.

## Case management systems

Several case management systems and various adaptations exist. And health care facilities continue to create new systems. But most facilities pattern their systems after the one developed at the New England Medical Center (NEMC), one of the first centers to use case management in an acute care setting. Facilities typically adapt this system to meet their own needs and philosophy of care.

## Tools for case management

Most facilities also pattern their case management tools after those used in the NEMC system. Called the case management plan and the critical path or health care map, these tools allow you to direct, evaluate, and revise patient progress and outcomes.

*Case management plan.* The basic tool of case management systems, the case management plan spells out the standardized care a patient with a specific DRG should receive. The plan covers:

• nursing-related problems
• patient outcomes
• intermediate patient outcomes
• nursing interventions
• medical interventions
• target times.

Each subsection of the plan covers a care unit the patient may be admitted to during his illness. For instance, a patient with a myocardial infarction may go to both the intensive care and medical-surgical units.

*Critical path.* Because of the length of case management plans, you probably won't use them on a daily basis. Instead, you'll turn to an ab-

breviated form of the plan: the critical path. The path covers only the key events that must occur for the patient to be discharged by the target date. Such events include consultations, diagnostic tests, physical activities the patient must perform, treatments, diet, medications, discharge planning, and patient teaching. (See *Following a critical path,* pages 116 and 117.)

If a standard critical path doesn't exist for a DRG you've had some experience with, you can develop one. In collaboration with a doctor who's also had experience with the DRG, outline the key events that must occur, taking into account the costs of resources and the expected length of stay. To adapt an existing path to a patient, you and the patient's primary doctor may need to modify some of the steps.

Once you've established a path, you must note any variances from it, grouping them by cause. Variances may result from the system, the caregivers, or a problem the patient develops, and they can be justifiable or not. For instance, you may have a patient who doesn't walk in the hall as scheduled. If he has a secondary infection that prevents him from walking, you'll list the variance as justifiable. But if the patient simply prefers to stay in bed watching television, you'll need to list the variance as not justifiable and take steps to correct the problem.

At shift report each day, you should review the critical paths with the other nurses. Before you go off duty, note any changes in the expected length of stay and point out critical events scheduled for the next shift to the nurses coming on duty. Also, discuss any variances that may have occurred during your shift.

## Drawbacks of case management

The case management system usually works well for a patient with one primary diagnosis, no secondary diagnoses, and few complications. But for some patients, you'll have trouble even establishing a time line. For instance, you can't easily predict when treatment will succeed for a patient with a seizure disorder. And for a patient with several variances, the expected course of treatment and length of stay will likely change, and documentation can become lengthy and complicated.

---

## Suggested readings

*Accreditation Manual for Hospitals.* Chicago: Joint Commission on Accreditation of Healthcare Organizations, 1991.

Del Togno-Armanasco, V., et al. "Developing an Integrated Nursing Case Management Model," *Nursing Management* 20(10):26-29, October 1989.

Dennison, P.D., and Keeling, A.W. "Clinical Support for Eliminating the Nursing Diagnosis of Knowledge Deficit," *Image: Journal of Nursing Scholarship* 21(3):142, Fall 1989.

Dolan, M. *Community and Home Health Care Plans.* Springhouse, Pa.: Springhouse Corp., 1989.

Etheredge, M.L., ed. *Collaborative Care: Nursing Care Management.* Chicago: American Hospital Publishing, Inc., 1989.

Holloway, N.M. *Medical-Surgical Care Plans.* Springhouse, Pa.: Springhouse Corp., 1988.

*Home Care Standards and Accreditation.* Chicago: Joint Commission on Accreditation of Healthcare Organizations, 1991.

Krenz, M., et al. "A Nursing Diagnosis Based Model: Guiding Nursing Practice," *Journal of Nursing Administration* 19(5):32-36, May 1989.

*Taxonomy I,* revised. St. Louis: North American Nursing Diagnosis Association, 1990.

Yura, H., and Walsh, M. *The Nursing Process,* 5th ed. Norwalk, Conn.: Appleton and Lange, 1988.

# 6

# NURSING INTERVENTION AND EVALUATION

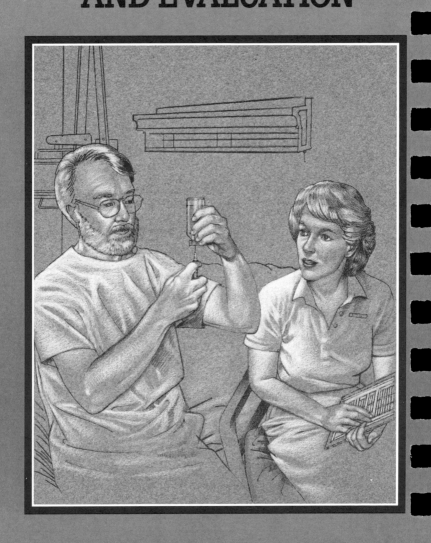

Documenting nursing interventions has long been standard practice. But documentation methods have changed dramatically over the years. No longer must you always write lengthy narrative notes. In many cases, you can use flow sheets or refer to a protocol instead.

The current emphasis on evaluating your interventions has also changed documentation. Today, your progress notes must include an assessment of your patient's progress toward the expected outcomes you've established in the care plan.

Perhaps the greatest change in documentation has been the development of new formats. Besides the traditional narrative and problem-oriented formats, you may also use such newer inventions as Focus charting, problem-intervention-evaluation (PIE) charting, and charting by exception (CBE).

This chapter will help you keep pace with these changes by explaining how to perform and document your interventions and evaluations. You'll find an entire section devoted to the different formats you may use to record interventions and evaluations. And you'll read how to document patient teaching and your patient's discharge summary.

# Performing your interventions and evaluations

Nursing intervention and evaluation represent crucial steps in the nursing process. When you carry out your interventions, you're putting your carefully constructed care plan into action. And when you

evaluate the results of your interventions, you help ensure that your plan is working.

## Interventions

Once you've established and recorded your care plan, you'll begin to implement it. You'll find that your interventions fall into two general categories: interdependent and independent. Before performing either type, you'll need to make a brief reassessment.

***Need for reassessment.*** Just before performing a particular intervention, you should quickly reassess the patient to ensure that your care plan remains appropriate. For example, what if the plan calls for helping the patient walk every 2 hours throughout the day, but your reassessment reveals that he recently returned from a physical therapy session and feels fatigued? In this case, making the patient walk would be inappropriate — despite the care plan.

***Types of interventions.*** Interdependent interventions include those you perform in collaboration with other health care professionals to help achieve a patient outcome. For example, if the outcome calls for the patient to walk independently on level surfaces, you'd support the physical therapist's regimen by reinforcing positioning and ambulation techniques between therapy sessions.

Interdependent interventions also include activities you perform at a doctor's request to help implement the medical regimen. These activities include administering medications and performing invasive procedures, such as indwelling urinary catheter insertion and venipuncture.

Independent interventions are

measures you take at your own discretion, independent of other health care team members. Such interventions include instituting common comfort measures and teaching routine self-care techniques.

**Evaluations**
In this phase of the nursing process, you'll compare the observed patient outcomes of your interventions with the expected outcomes established during the planning phase. Evaluation consists of three steps:
• referring to a specific standard—for example, an outcome statement such as "Lose 2 lb by 1/9/92"
• noting relevant information—for example, a weight loss of 2¼ lb by 1/9/92.
• making a judgment in light of the data—for example, "Outcome was achieved."

*When to evaluate.* Evaluation itself is an ongoing process that takes place whenever you see your patient. But how often you're required to make evaluations will be influenced by several factors, including where you work. If you work in an acute care setting, your facility's policy may require you to review care plans every 24 hours. But if you work in a long-term care facility, the required interval between evaluations may be up to 30 days. In either case, this doesn't mean that you shouldn't evaluate and revise the care plan more often, if warranted.
How often you make your evaluations may also be influenced by the specific interventions in the plan. For instance, interventions for an unstable patient in an intensive care unit would require frequent evaluation.

*What follows evaluation.* After an

outcome has been achieved, you and the patient may decide that the pertinent nursing diagnosis no longer applies. In this case, you'd document which outcome has been met and how, then delete the diagnosis from the care plan in accordance with your facility's policy.
Alternately, you and the patient may deem a goal met, according to the outcome criteria, but decide that the nursing diagnosis remains valid and that interventions are still needed. For example, when a short-term outcome of a 2-lb weight loss per week has been met but the long-term outcome of a 30-lb weight loss hasn't yet been achieved, the original nursing diagnosis remains valid.
An unmet or partially met outcome requires that you review the available data and the nursing care plan. In some cases, your review may reveal an omission in the plan or a misinterpretation of the data. For example, if your patient didn't lose 2 lb as expected, the review may indicate that the patient needs more information on nutrition (omission). Or the patient may have a premenstrual weight gain (misinterpretation).
After identifying any omissions or misinterpretations, revise the care plan. This may involve the following:
• clarifying or amending the data base to reflect newly discovered information
• reexamining and correcting nursing diagnoses
• establishing outcome criteria that reflect new information and new or amended nursing strategies
• adding this revised nursing care plan to the original document
• recording the rationale for the revisions in the nurses' progress notes.

# Documenting your interventions and evaluations

You need to record the fact that you performed an intervention, the time you performed it, the patient's response to it, and any other interventions that you took based on his response. You should also include your reasons for these additional interventions. And for all interventions, you need to include your evaluation of the outcome. (See *Charting patient responses.*) Recording all this information makes your documentation outcome-oriented.

You can document interventions on graphic records, a patient care flowsheet that integrates all nurses' notes for a 1-day period, integrated or separate nurses' progress notes, and other specialized documentation forms, such as the medication administration record (MAR). In most cases, you'll document your evaluations in your progress notes. Your facility's policies will dictate the exact style, format, and location of your documentation. You'll record interventions and evaluations when you give routine care, observe changes in the patient's condition, give emergency care, and administer medications.

## Routine care
For years, the Joint Commission on Accreditation of Healthcare Organizations (JCAHO) has encouraged health care facilities to use flow sheets for documenting routine care measures. In response, many facilities have developed these forms for such measures as making basic assessments, giving wound care, and

## Charting patient responses

When documenting your evaluations, remember to include your patient's responses to the following:
☐ administration of medications given as needed
☐ changes in or progression of activity
☐ changes in or progression of diet
☐ patient education
☐ treatments (nursing and medical)
☐ unusual incidents
☐ discharge plans.

providing hygiene. In many facilities, you may also use flow sheets to document vital signs checks, intravenous monitoring, equipment checks, patient education, and discharge summaries. (See *Using a flow sheet for routine care*, pages 124 to 127.)

You'll see various flow sheet formats. Some are simple patient care checklists. Others provide space for you to record specific care given. Some even provide space for evaluative statements.

Because of their brevity, flow sheets make documenting and reviewing documented material quick and easy. Specifically, they allow you to evaluate patient trends at a glance. But keep in mind that overusing flow sheets can lead to fragmented documentation that may obscure the patient's clinical picture.

## Changes in condition
In your progress notes, you'll need to document any changes in your patient's condition. Suppose, for instance, that you observe a sudden increase in your patient's wound

*(Text continues on page 128.)*

CHARTING

## Using a flow sheet for routine care

As this sample shows, a patient care flow sheet allows you to quickly document your routine interventions. Note that the last page of this 4-page form provides space for narrative notes.

**PATIENT CARE FLOW SHEET**

| Date 1/22/92 | 11 p.m. - 7 a.m. | 7 a.m. - 3 p.m. | 3 p.m. - 11 p.m. |
|---|---|---|---|
| **RESPIRATORY** | | | |
| Lung sounds | CLEAR 12 AG | Crackles ®Ant.#9 chest BAL | Clear 4:30 BB 10 BB |
| Treatments/results | — | Nebulizer 10:30* BAL | — |
| Cough/results | ō AG | Lg. amount 10:30 thick white mucus BAL | sm. amt. thin, clear mucus 7:30 BB |
| O₂ therapy Nasal cannula @ 2L/min | CONTINUOUS AG | with activity 108AL Pulse 90 with activity 2 BAL Pulse 88 | with activity 7 BB pulse 92 with activity 9 BB pulse 96 |
| **CARDIAC** | | | |
| Chest pain | ō AG | ō BAL | ō BB |
| Heart sounds | NORMAL S₁ AND S₂ AG | Normal heart sounds BAL | normal S₁ and S₂ BB |
| Telemetry | N/A | N/A | n/a |
| **PAIN** | | | |
| Type & location | SL. ABDOMINAL 2 AG | Abdominal 10 BAL | abdominal 7:30 BB |
| Intervention | VOIDED AG | Percocet + repositioning BAL | Tylenol - backrub BB |
| Response | IMMEDIATE IMPROVEMENT AG | Improved from #8 to #3 in ½ hr BAL | Complete relief in 1 hr BB |
| **NUTRITION** | | | |
| Type | — | Regular | Regular |
| Toleration % | — | 100% | 50% |
| Supplement | — | — BAL | Soup from home BB |
| **ELIMINATION** | | | |
| Stool appearance | ī/ō AG | ī/ Light brown 11 BAL | ī/ō BB |
| Enema | N/A | N/A | n/a |
| Results | ↓ | ↓ | ↓ |
| Bowel sounds | PRESENT 12 AG | Present all quadrants 9 BAL | Present 4:30 BB |

**PATIENT CARE FLOW SHEET** page 2

| Date 1/22/92 | 11 p.m. - 7 a.m. | 7 a.m. - 3 p.m. | 3 p.m. - 11 p.m. |
|---|---|---|---|
| **ELIMINATION** (continued) | | | |
| Urine appearance | CLEAR AMBER 2 AG | Light yellow 1 BAL | Clear amber 7 BB |
| | | | |
| Foley catheter | N/A | N/A | n/a |
| Catheter irrigations | | | |
| | ↓ | ↓ | ↓ |
| **I.V. THERAPY** | | | |
| Tubing change | — | | |
| Dressing change | — | | |
| Site appearance | NO EDEMA 12 AG | non-reddened/no drainage 10 BAL | Clean — 9 BB no edema |
| **WOUND** | | | |
| Type | Ⓛ LEG | Ⓛ lower leg | Ⓛ leg |
| Dressing change | DRESSINGS DRY 12AG 6AG | 11:30 * BAL | 7:30 * BB |
| Appearance | WOUND NOT OBSERVED AG | 3"L×¼"W. lg amt. pink-yellow drainage 11:30 BAL | mod. amt. yellow drainage 7:30 BB |
| Irrigate b.i.d. | | 11:30 BAL | 7:30 ē diluted H₂O₂ solution BB |
| **TUBES** | | | |
| Type | N/A | N/A | n/a |
| Irrigation | | | |
| Drainage appearance | ↓ | ↓ | ↓ |
| **HYGIENE** | | | |
| Self/partial/complete | — | Partial 10:30 BAL | Partial 9 VG |
| Oral care | — | 10:30 BAL | 9 VG |
| Back care | — | 10:30 BAL | 7:30 VG |
| Foot care | — | 10:30 BAL | — |
| Remove/reapply elastic stockings rt. leg | 12 AG | 10:30 BAL | 9 VG |

(continued)

CHARTING

## Using a flow sheet for routine care *(continued)*

**PATIENT CARE FLOW SHEET**                                                                  page 3

| Date 1/22/92 | 11 p.m. - 7 a.m. | 7 a.m. - 3 p.m. | 3 p.m. - 11 p.m. |
|---|---|---|---|
| **ACTIVITY** | | | |
| Type | BEDREST    AG | Dangle legs x10 min 2:30 BAL | Stand at bedside x5 min    BB |
| Toleration | TURNS SELF    AG | Sl. dizziness BP 110/70 BAL | Initial dizziness BP lying 120/84 Stand 116/70 BB |
| Repositioned | 12    AG | Back -8 BAL 12 BAL ®side 10 BAL 2 BAL | Self    BB |
| ROM | — | 10:30 (passive) 2 BAL BAL (active) | 6 BB (active) 9 VG (active) |
| **SLEEP** | | | |
| Sleeps well | 4 AG  6 AG | N/A | n/a |
| Awake at intervals | 12 AG  2 AG | ↓ | ↓ |
| Awake most of the time | — — | | |
| **SAFETY** | | | |
| Side rails up | 12AG 2AG 4AG 6AG | 8 BAL    2:30 BAL | 6 BB    9 VG |
| Call light in reach | 12 AG    4 AG | 8 BAL    12 BAL | 4 BB 6 BB 11 BB |
| **EQUIPMENT** | | | |
| Type 1-med pump | CONTINUOUS 12 AG | continuous 8 BAL | continuous 4 BB |
| | | | |
| | | | |
| | | | |
| **TEACHING** | | | |
| Breathing exercises | | 10:30 BAL | |
| NPO before upper GI | | | 4:30* BB |
| | | | |
| | | | |
| | | | |
| | | | |

**PATIENT CARE FLOW SHEET** page 4

### PROGRESS SHEET

| Time | Comments |
|---|---|
| 9 a.m. | Dr. Jones notified re crackles and Pt.'s inability to cough. Skin pale, respirations 32, shallow. Nebulizer treatment ordered. ———— *Barbara A. Lane, RN* |
| 10:30 a.m. | Skin color improved following successful nebulizer Rx. Lungs clear, respirations 20. Reviewed pursed lip and abdominal breathing techniques. Pt. indicated he had been taught this before but forgets to do it. Demonstrated pursed lip breathing correctly, but needs further practice on abdominal breathing. ———— *Barbara A. Lane, RN* |
| 11:30 a.m. | During dressing change and irrigation changed to 1:1 solution $H_2O_2$ and sterile saline. *Barbara A. Lane, RN* |
| 7:30 p.m. | ⊕ leg dressing and irrigation completed using diluted solution. No further reports of discomfort. Pt. noted using pursed lip breathing during position changes. *Barbara Black, RN* |
| 9:00 p.m. | Pt. instructed in expectations re U.G.I. earlier. Pt. related correct understanding of test purpose and procedure. Has had nothing to eat or drink since 8 p.m. ———— *Barbara Black, RN* |
| | |
| | |
| | |

| INITIALS | SIGNATURE/TITLE |
|---|---|
| AG | Alice Gray RN |
| BAL | Barbara A. Lane, RN |
| BB | Barbara Black, RN |
| VG | Vicki Grove, LPN |

drainage. In a narrative format, your progress note describing this observation should look something like this:

12/5/91, 11 a.m. Left arm wound drainage has saturated six 4″ × 4″ gauze pads and one 4″ × 8″ dressing since last dressing check at 10 a.m. Wound dimensions remain as on 12/4 note, but drainage now dark yellow and foul-smelling. Obtained specimens for culture and sensitivity testing and sent to the lab per impaired skin integrity protocol. Cleaned wound with hydrogen peroxide. (See care plan for dressing change orders.) Patient states, "My arm is really throbbing." Administered Darvon-N and repositioned patient to semi-Fowler's position with left arm supported on pillow.

This example refers to a protocol or standard of care for patients with a nursing diagnosis of impaired skin integrity. Because this protocol mandates cleaning with hydrogen peroxide and culture and sensitivity testing for a patient with purulent wound drainage, no further doctor's orders or clarification is required.

The note also directs readers to the patient's care plan for specific dressing change methods. The reader would also know to check the MAR for specific information about the pain medication given.

The note goes on to specify information about the other pain relief measure implemented as well as the patient's comments about the pain's characteristics. And it doesn't repeat information recorded elsewhere in the chart, so it's concise yet informative.

**Emergency situations**

When documenting a patient emergency (for example, a cardiac ar-

rest), follow standard guidelines, taking care to:
• be factual.
• be specific about times and interventions.
• include the name of the doctor you contacted, when you contacted him, and what you told him.
• indicate attempts to inform the patient's family or significant others of the changes in his situation.

Look at the following sample for tips on how to document an emergency situation:

1/23/92, 9 p.m. Was summoned to the patient's room at 8:20 p.m. by a shout from roommate. Found patient unresponsive, without respirations or pulse. Roommate stated, "He was talking to me, then all of a sudden started gasping and holding his chest." Called a code and, along with J. Prince, RN, initiated CPR. Code team arrived at 8:25 and continued resuscitation efforts (see code record). Patient eventually stabilized and opened his eyes. Notified Dr. Jones at his home at 8:40 and explained situation; he said he'll be in to see patient immediately. Telephoned patient's wife at home at 8:50 and told her of his changed condition and his imminent transfer to ICU. She said she'll return to the hospital as soon as she can.

In this sample, note the reference to the code record. This specialized documentation form incorporates detailed information about a code, including observations, interventions, and medications administered. (See *Using a code record.*) Using this reference keeps the progress note concise, while ensuring complete documentation.

**Medication administration**

Most health care facilities have in-

CHARTING

## Using a code record

This sample shows the typical features of a code record.

### CODE RECORD

Name _Roy Walden_      Body weight _165 lb_    Date _1/23/92_

| Time a.m. (p.m.) | BP | Heart rate | Heart rhythm | Atropine (mg) | Calcium chloride (ampules) | Epinephrine (mg) | Lidocaine (mg) | Procainamide (mg) | Sodium bicarb (ampules) | Dopamine (mg/ml) | Isoproterenol (mg/ml) | Lidocaine (g/ml) | Defibrillation (joules) | CPR | Airway | PaO₂ | PaCO₂ | HCO₃⁻ | pH |
|---|---|---|---|---|---|---|---|---|---|---|---|---|---|---|---|---|---|---|---|
| | | | | **Bolus meds** | | | | | | **Infused meds** | | | **Actions** | | | **Blood gases** | | | |
| 8:20 | 0 | 0 | | | | | | | | | | | | ✓ | mask | | | | |
| 8:25 | 0 | 0 | VF | | | | | | | | | | | | | | | | |
| 8:25 | | | | | | | | | | | | | 200 | | | | | | |
| 8:26 | | | | | | | | | | | | | | ✓ | | | | | |
| 8:27 | | | | | | | | | | | | | 300 | | | | | | |
| 8:29 | | | | | | | | | | | | | 360 | | | | | | |
| 8:30 | | | | | | | 1 | 75 | | | | | | ✓ | ET tube | 27 | 76 | 14 | 7.10 |
| 8:31 | | | | | | | | | | | | | 360 | | | | | | |
| 8:31 | | | ↓ | | | | | 1 | | | | | | ✓ | | | | | |
| 8:32 | | NSR | | | | | | | | | | | 360 | | | | | | |
| 8:32 | | NSR | | | | | | | | | | | | | | | | | |
| 8:35 | 140/90 | 96 | ↓ | | | | | 75 | | | | | | | | 43 | 26 | 23 | 7.46 |

**Time    Actions**

8:20 Code called. CPR initiated by E. Land, RN, and J. Prince, RN.
8:20 Bagged by J. Prince, RN.
8:25 Single-channel ECG. Central line inserted via Ⓛ subclavian by Dr. Kee.
8:29 ABG via Ⓡ femoral artery by Dr. Jay. Oral intubation by anesthesiologist.
8:32 Converted to NSR.
8:35 ABG via Ⓛ femoral artery. Pressure applied. Unresponsive.

Time code called _8:20_
☐ Arrest witnessed
☑ Arrest unwitnessed
☑ Intubation _8:29_
☑ Arrhythmia _V-Fib_
☑ Informed family
☑ Informed attending doctor

Disposition
☐ SICU
☑ MICU
☐ CCU
☐ OR
☐ Morgue
☐ Other

Status after resuscitation
BP 140/90
Heart rate 96. Bagged with
100% O₂ and transported
to MICU.

Critical care nurse
_D. Sayer, RN_

Code chief _W. Kee, MD_

corporated some type of MAR into their documentation system. Commonly contained in a Kardex file or on a separate medication administration sheet, the MAR serves as the central source for recording the medication orders and for documenting their execution. The MAR becomes part of the patient's permanent record.

When using a MAR, keep these guidelines in mind:
• Know and follow your facility's policies and procedures for recording medication orders and charting medication administration.
• Make sure all medication orders include the patient's full name, the date, name of the drug, dose, administration route or method, and frequency. Make sure the time of a stat dose is indicated. When appropriate, include the specific number of doses or the stop date.
• Write legibly.
• Use only standard abbreviations and use them correctly. When in doubt as to how to abbreviate a term, spell it out.
• After administering the first dose, sign your full name, licensure status, and your initials in the appropriate space on the MAR.

If you work in a health care facility that charts medications by computer, input your information for each drug right after you give it. This is particularly important if you don't use printouts as a backup. By keying in information immediately, you ensure that all health care team members have access to up-to-the-minute medication data.

If you administer all medications according to the care plan, you don't need any further documentation. However, if your facility's MAR doesn't include space to document such aspects as parenteral administration site, the patient's response

to medications given as needed, or any deviations from the medication order, you'll need to include narrative documentation in your progress notes.

# Documenting within a format

Various formats have been developed in an effort to promote efficiency and fulfill current requirements. Depending on the policies of the health care facility where you work, you'll use one or more of the following five formats to document your interventions and evaluations. As you'll see, these formats also cover your assessments, but their primary focus is intervention and evaluation. (See *Comparing documentation formats.*)

### Traditional narrative format
In this paragraph approach to charting, you document ongoing assessment data, nursing interventions, and patient responses in chronological order. You'll record this information in your nurses' progress notes. Today, few facilities use only the narrative format. Most also use flow sheets to save time. (See *Using the narrative format*, page 132.)

***Better narrative documentation.*** You can improve your narrative documentation by knowing when to document, what to document, and how to organize your notes.

*When to document.* Current JCAHO standards direct all health care facilities to establish policies on the frequency of patient reassessment. So you must assess your patient at

## Comparing documentation formats

| BENEFITS | NARRATIVE | PROBLEM-ORIENTED | FOCUS | PIE | CHARTING BY EXCEPTION |
|---|---|---|---|---|---|
| Promotes use of nursing process, including nursing diagnosis and evaluation of outcomes | N | S | A | A | S |
| Provides organizational structure for notes | N | A | A | A | A |
| Saves time | N | N | A | S | A |
| Improves clarity | N | S | A | A | A |
| Facilitates data retrieval | N | A | A | A | A |
| Fulfills JCAHO requirements | S | S | A | S | A |

**KEY:**
A = Always
S = Sometimes
N = Never

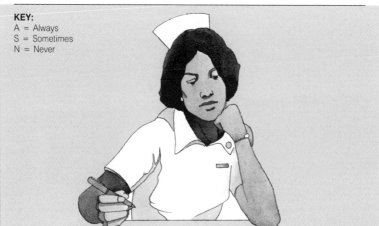

least as often as required by your facility's policy, then document your findings.

The problem with charting too often is that you may find yourself writing repetitious, meaningless notes. If this occurs, double-check your facility's policy. You may find that you're following a time-consuming, unwritten standard that staff members have initiated, rather than the written policy. To guard against this, review your facility's policy at least every 6 months. (See *When to write narrative notes*, page 134.)

*What to document.* Document exactly what you've heard, observed, inspected, done, or taught. Include

## Using the narrative format

This sample shows how to write a progress note using the narrative format.

PROGRESS SHEET

| Date | Time | Comments |
|------|------|----------|
| 1/22/92 | 10 a.m. | Observed Ⓛ lower leg wound 3" long x ¼" wide x ¼" deep; three 4"x 4" gauze pads saturated with pink-yellow nonodorous drainage; surrounding skin reddened and tender. Redressed wound with four 4"x 4"s and one 4"x8" dressing and non-allergenic tape. Will check wound q 1 hr to assess for continued drainage and signs of infection. Pt. reports pain in Ⓛ leg at 8 on a scale of 1 to 10. Administered Percocet and repositioned from back to Ⓡ side. Will give Percocet ½ hour before subsequent dressing change. Instructed pt. in dressing change procedure. Pt. stated "I know that it's important to wash my hands before I do anything so I don't get germs in my wound." Pt. demonstrates sufficient manual dexterity to put on gloves and handle all dressing supplies. Instructed pt. in proper hand-washing technique, dressing removal and disposal, opening and positioning of dressing supplies, signs and symptoms of wound infection and the importance of reporting them. Pt. demonstrated acceptable hand-washing technique and ability to remove dressings, but needed instruction on positioning the leg so she could reach the wound. (Continued on next page.) —Barbara A. Lene, RN |

as much specific, descriptive information as possible. For example, if your patient has lower leg edema, include ankle and mid-calf measurements as well as skin characteristics. Always document how the patient has responded to your care and the extent to which he's progressing toward the desired outcomes.

Here are a few simple suggestions that can help you write meaningful narrative notes:

• Read the notes written by other health care professionals before you write your own.

• Read the notes recorded by nurses on other shifts and make further comments on their findings to demonstrate continuity of care.

• If policy permits, use flow sheets to document repetitious procedures or measurements and summarize the information in the narrative note.

• Be sure to include specific information when you observe a change in your patient's condition, a lack of progress in his condition, a response to treatment or medication, or a response to patient teaching.

*Organization tips.* Before you write anything, organize your thoughts so your paragraphs will be coherent. If you have difficulty deciding what to say in your notes, refer to the patient's care plan to review unresolved problems, expected outcomes, and prescribed interventions. Then comment on the patient's progress in relation to these items.

If you still have trouble organizing your thoughts, try following this sequence of questions:

• How did I first become aware of the problem?

• What has the patient said that's significant about the problem?

• What have I observed that's related to the problem?

• What's my plan for dealing with the problem?

• What steps have I taken to intervene?

• How has the patient responded to my interventions?

To make your notes as coherent as possible, discuss each of the patient's problems in a separate paragraph; don't lump them all together.

*Advantages.* Traditional narrative notes have a couple of advantages. Because narration is the most common form of writing, proper use of narrative notes usually requires little training time for new staff members. The format also provides an easy way to document information collected over an extended period.

*Disadvantages.* With the narrative format, tracking problems and trends in the patient's progress can be difficult. Because the format offers no inherent guide to what's important to document, notes may tend to become long, rambling, and repetitive. The narrative format also lends itself to vague or inaccurate language — for example, phrases such as "appears to be bleeding" or "small amount."

## Problem-oriented format

The problem-oriented medical record (POMR) system, sometimes known as the problem-oriented record (POR) system, focuses on specific patient problems. With this format, you'll describe each problem on multidisciplinary patient progress notes, not on progress notes containing only nursing information. This format allows better coordination and communication among team members and promotes a more comprehensive, coordinated approach to planning and documenting care.

# When to write narrative notes

Typically, you should document using narrative notes when you observe any of the following:

☐ a change in the patient's condition (progression, regression, or new problems). Be specific in describing the change. For example, say, "The patient can walk the length of the hall with the assistance of one person."

☐ a patient's response to a treatment or medication. For example, you might write, "The patient states that left leg pain is unrelieved 1 hour after receiving medication. He's still grimacing and rubbing the site."

☐ a lack of improvement in the patient's condition. For example, say, "No change in size or condition of leg wound after 5 days of treatment. Dimensions and condition remain as stated in 12/15/91 note."

☐ a patient's or family member's response to teaching. For example, you'd note, "The patient performed a return demonstration of wound care and correctly stated that it was to be done three times a day."

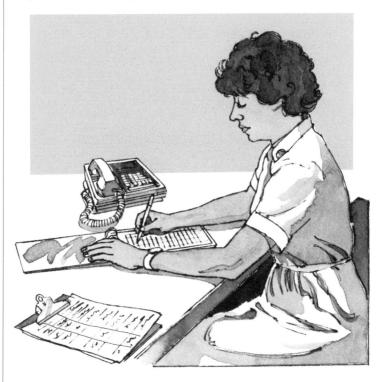

(See *Using the problem-oriented format*, page 136.)

**POMR components.** The POMR consists of five components: data base, problem list, initial plan, progress notes, and discharge summary. You'll record your interventions and evaluations in the progress notes and the discharge summary only. But to gain a full understanding of the POMR, briefly review all five components.

*Data base.* Most commonly completed by a nurse, the data base (or initial assessment) forms the foundation for the patient's care plan. As discussed in Chapter 4, the initial assessment includes such information as the reason for hospitalization, allergies, medication regimen, physical and psychosocial findings, self-care ability, educational needs, and other discharge planning concerns.

*Problem list.* After analyzing the data base, you, the doctor, and possibly other health care team members will identify and list the patient's current problems in chronologic order according to the date each was identified — not in order of acuteness or priority. Originally, this system called for one interdisciplinary problem list. You may still see this format used, but usually nurses and doctors keep separate problem lists, with problems stated as either nursing or medical diagnoses.

Each problem should be numbered, so you can use the numbers to refer to the problems in the rest of the POMR. To do so, make every entry on the patient's initial plan, progress notes, and discharge summary correspond to a number, and file the numbered problem list at the front of the patient's chart. Keep the problem list current by adding new numbers as new problems arise. Once a problem has been resolved, draw a line through it or show that it's inactive by drawing a line over it and its number with a yellow highlighter. Don't use that number again for the same patient.

*Initial plan.* After drawing up the problem list, you'll write an initial plan for each problem. This plan should include the expected outcomes, plans for further data collection (if needed), and treatment and patient education plans.

*Progress notes.* One of the most prominent features of the POMR system is the structured way in which narrative progress notes are written by all team members, using the SOAP or SOAPIE format. If you use the SOAP format, you'll document the following information for each problem:
S = Subjective data: information the patient tells you
O = Objective data: factual data you gather during assessment
A = Assessment: conclusions you reach about the patient's problem based on the subjective and objective information
P = Plan: your plan to relieve the patient's problem.
   Some facilities use the SOAPIE format, adding:
I = Intervention: measures you've taken to achieve a patient outcome
E = Evaluation: an analysis of whether your interventions were effective.
   Typically, you must write a complete SOAP or SOAPIE note every 24 hours on any unresolved problem or whenever the patient's condition changes. When doing so, be sure to specify the appropriate number of

CHARTING

## Using the problem-oriented format

This sample shows how to write a progress note using the problem-oriented format.

PROGRESS SHEET

| Date | Time | Comments |
|------|------|----------|
| 1/22/92 | 10 a.m. | #1 Impaired skin integrity R/T leg wound |
| | | S: "my dressing is leaking." |
| | | O: ⓛ lower leg wound 3" long x ¼" wide x ¼" deep; three 4"x4" gauze pads saturated with pink-yellow nonodorous drainage; surrounding skin not reddened. |
| | | A: Drainage increased over the past 4hr |
| | | P: Increase dressing to four 4"x4" pads and one 4"x8" dressing with nonallergenic tape. Check dressing q1hr to assess for continued drainage increase, and assess for signs of infection at each dressing change. ———— Barbara A. Lane, RN |
| | 10 a.m. | #2 Pain R/T ⓛ leg wound |
| | | S: Pt. reports pain at 8 on a scale of 1 to 10. |
| | | O: Wound site as described above. Pt. grimacing and pointing to leg. BP 130/84 pulse 96. |
| | | A: Existing pain aggravated by dressing change. Vital signs increased over baseline; see graphic record. |
| | | P: Administer Percocet. Reposition pt. from back to Ⓡ side. Assess pain relief in 1 hr and administer Percocet ½ hr before subsequent dressing changes. ———— Barbara A. Lane, RN |
| 1/22/92 | 11 a.m. | #2 Pain R/T ⓛ leg wound |
| | | S: Pt. states pain now a 3 on a scale of 1 to 10 and that this is acceptable to her. |
| | | O: Pt. looks relaxed. Able to reposition (continued on next page.) Barbara A. Lane, RN |

the problem you're discussing. Keep in mind that you don't need to write an entry for each SOAP or SOAPIE component every time you document. If you have nothing to record for a component, either omit the letter from the note or leave a blank space after it, depending on your facility's policy.

If your facility uses the SOAP format, you'll record your nursing interventions and evaluations on flow sheets. If you use the SOAPIE format, you'll provide explanations as needed in your progress notes under I and E.

*Discharge summary.* Completing the POMR format, the discharge summary covers each problem on the list and notes whether or not it was resolved. Discuss any unresolved problems in your SOAP or SOAPIE note, specifying your plans for solving the problem after discharge. Note any communications with other facilities, home care agencies, and the patient.

**Advantages.** The POMR organizes information about each problem into specific categories understandable to all team members, thus promoting interdisciplinary communication. The POMR also unifies the care plan and progress notes into a complete record of care actually planned and delivered. And this format promotes documentation of the nursing process, facilitates more consistent documentation, and eliminates documentation of nonessential data.

**Disadvantages.** The POMR also has several disadvantages. Simply listing the problems in chronologic order can make it difficult to determine the priority problems. The format can also make analyzing trends difficult because information is buried in daily narrative notes.

This format commonly produces repetitious charting of assessment findings and interventions, especially with the SOAPIE format. That's because both your assessments and interventions frequently apply to more than one problem. The resulting overlap makes this method time-consuming.

## Focus charting format

Developed by nurses who found the SOAP format awkward, Focus charting encourages you to organize your thoughts into patient-centered topics, or foci of concern, and then to document precisely and concisely. The format encourages you to use assessment data to evaluate these patient care concerns. It also helps you identify necessary revisions to the care plan as you document each entry.

**Documentation process.** This format has columns for the date, time, focus, and progress notes. (See *Using the Focus charting format*, page 138.)

*Documenting the focus.* You'll identify foci by reviewing the assessment data. Typically, you'll write each focus as a nursing diagnosis. However, the focus may also refer to a sign or symptom (for example, hypotension), a patient behavior or special need (such as discharge needs), an acute change in the patient's condition (loss of consciousness, for example), or a significant event (such as surgery).

*Data-action-response.* In the progress notes column, you'll organize information using three categories: data (D), action (A), and response (R). In the data category, you'll include subjective and objective infor-

CHARTING

## Using the Focus charting format

This sample shows how to write progress notes using the Focus charting format.

### PROGRESS SHEET

| Date | Time | Focus | Progress notes |
|------|------|-------|----------------|
| 1/22/92 | 10 a.m. | Impaired skin integrity R/T Ⓛ leg wound | D: Ⓛ lower leg wound 3" long × ¼" wide × ¼" deep; three 4"× 4" gauze pads saturated with pink-yellow nonodorous drainage; surrounding skin not reddened or tender. ————— <br> A: Wound redressed with four 4"×4" gauze pads and one 4"×8" dressing and nonallergenic tape. (See care plan.) Will check wound q1 hr to assess for continued drainage increase and signs of infection. <br> ————————— Barbara A. Lane, RN |
| 1/22/92 | 10 a.m. | Pain R/T Ⓛ leg wound | D: Pt. reports pain in Ⓛ lower leg at 8 on scale of 1 to 10. Wound site as described above. ————— <br> A: Administered Percocet and repositioned from back to Ⓡ side. Will administer Percocet ½ hr before all subsequent dressing changes. (See care plan.) Barbara A. Lane, RN |
| | 10 a.m. | Pt. teaching | Pt. states, "I know that it's important to wash my hands before I do anything so I don't get any germs in my wound." Pt. demonstrates sufficient manual dexterity to put on gloves and handle all dressing supplies. <br> A: Instructed pt. in proper hand-washing technique, dressing removal and disposal, opening and positioning of dressing supplies, and the signs and symptoms of wound infection and the importance of reporting them. <br> R: Pt. demonstrates acceptable handwashing technique and ability to remove dressing, but (Continued on next page.) Barbara Lane, RN |

mation that describes the focus. The action category should include immediate and future nursing actions based on your assessment of the situation. This category also may encompass any changes to the care plan you deem necessary, based on your evaluation. Under the response category, you'll describe the patient's response to any aspect of nursing or medical care.

Using all three categories ensures complete documentation based on the nursing process. Be sure to record routine nursing tasks and assessment data on your flow sheets and checklists.

**Advantages.** By keeping the focus statement separate from the body of the progress note, this format makes it easy to find information on a particular problem, thus facilitating communication among health care team members. The format also highlights the nursing process in the documentation of daily patient care, encourages regular documentation of patient responses to nursing and medical therapy, and ensures adherence to JCAHO requirements for documenting patient responses and outcomes.

You can use this format to document many topics without being confined to those on the problem list or care plan. You also may find that the format helps you organize your thoughts and document more succinctly and precisely.

**Disadvantages.** The Focus charting system may call for in-depth training for staff members used to other documentation systems. Also, to use this system properly, you need many flow sheets and checklists. This can lead to inconsistent documentation and cause difficulty in tracking a patient's problems.

## Problem-intervention-evaluation format

Developed to simplify the documentation process, problem-intervention-evaluation (PIE) charting organizes information based on patient problems. As the name indicates, this problem-oriented approach uses three documentation categories: problem (P), intervention (I), and evaluation (E). Documentation tools for this format include a daily patient assessment flow sheet and progress notes.

By integrating the care plan into the nurses' progress notes, the PIE format eliminates the need for a separate care plan. The intention is to provide a concise, efficient record of patient care that has a nursing — not a medical — focus. (See *Using the PIE format,* page 140.)

**Documentation process.** You'll begin the process by assessing the patient and documenting your findings on a daily patient assessment flow sheet. This flow sheet lists defined assessment terms under major categories, such as respiration, along with routine care and monitoring such as providing hygiene and monitoring lung sounds. The form also typically includes space to record pertinent treatments. On the form, you'll initial only those assessment terms that apply to your patient and mark abnormal findings with an asterisk. Detailed information goes in your progress notes.

*Problem.* After performing and documenting an initial assessment, use the data to identify pertinent nursing diagnoses. You can use the list of nursing diagnoses accepted by your facility, usually the diagnoses approved by the North American Nursing Diagnosis Association (NANDA). If you can't find a

CHARTING

## Using the PIE format

This sample shows how to write progress notes using the problem-intervention-evaluation (PIE) format.

### PROGRESS SHEET

| Date | Time | Comments |
|------|------|----------|
| 1/22/92 | 10 a.m. | P#1: Impaired skin integrity R/T ⓛ lower leg wound. |
| | | I P#1: Dressing change; dressings increased to four 4"×4" gauze pads and one 4"×8" dressing because of increased drainage. |
| | | EP #1: Drainage increased; saturated previous dressing of three 4"×4" pads. Wound dimensions stable. Will monitor drainage amount and characteristics carefully. ——— Barbara A. Lane, RN |
| 1/22/92 | 10 a.m. | P#2: Pain R/T ⓛ lower leg wound |
| | | I P#2: Administered Percocet and repositioned pt. from back to ⓡ side. Provided back rub. |
| | | EP #2: Existing pain aggravated by dressing change. Vital signs increased over baseline. Will give Percocet for pain ½ hr before dressing changes. ——— Barbara A. Lane, RN |
| 1/22/92 | 11 a.m. | EP#2: Pt. reports pain reduced from 8 to 3 on a scale of 1 to 10. Pt. states this is acceptable. ——— Barbara A. Lane, RN |

nursing diagnosis on an approved list, write the problem statement yourself using accepted criteria.

Document all nursing diagnoses or problems in the progress notes, labeling each as "P" with an identifying number (for example, P #1). This labeling system allows you to refer to a specific problem in the future by label only, eliminating the need to redocument the problem statement. Some facilities also use a separate problem list form to keep a convenient running list of the nursing diagnoses for a particular patient.

*Intervention.* In this step, you document the nursing actions taken for each nursing diagnosis. Document interventions on the progress notes, labeling each as "I" followed by the assigned problem number. To refer to an intervention for the first nursing diagnosis, for instance, you'd use IP #1.

*Evaluation.* After charting your interventions, document the related outcomes in your progress notes. Use the label "E," followed by the assigned problem number — for example, EP #1.

Make sure that you or another nurse evaluates each problem at least every 8 hours. After every three shifts, review the notes from the previous 24 hours to identify the patient's current problems and responses to interventions. Document continuing problems daily, along with relevant interventions and evaluations. Cross out any resolved problems from the daily documentation.

**Advantages.** Using the PIE format ensures that your documentation identifies your nursing diagnoses, related interventions, and evalua-

tions. This format also encourages you to meet JCAHO requirements, provides a framework to help organize your thoughts and writing, and simplifies documentation by incorporating your plan of care into your nurses' progress notes.

**Disadvantages.** Like the Focus charting system, the PIE format may require in-depth training for staff members. And the requirement that you reevaluate each problem each shift leads to repetitive charting; some problems simply don't need such frequent evaluation.

## Charting by exception format
The charting by exception (CBE) format was designed to overcome longstanding problems in documentation. These include lengthy and repetitive notes, poorly organized information, difficult-to-retrieve data, and a high risk of errors. To avoid these pitfalls, the CBE format radically departs from traditional systems by requiring documentation of *only* significant or abnormal findings. It also uses military time to help prevent misinterpretations.

To use the CBE format effectively, you must know and adhere to established guidelines for nursing assessments and interventions. The CBE nursing assessment format has printed guidelines for each body system. Guidelines for interventions are derived from these sources:
• nursing diagnoses-based standardized care plans. These plans identify patient problems, desired outcomes, and planned interventions.
• protocols. These guidelines consist of standardized interventions established for care of specific patient populations — for example, patients with a nursing diagnosis of pain.
• doctor's orders. These are prescribed medical interventions.

• incidental orders. These are typically one-time, miscellaneous nursing or medical orders or interdependent interventions related to a protocol or a piece of equipment.
• standards of nursing practice. These standards define the minimum level of routine nursing care for all patients. They may be hospital- or unit-based.

**Documentation tools.** The CBE format involves a care plan and several types of flow sheets, including the nursing-medical order flow sheet, graphic record, patient-teaching record, and patient discharge note. In certain cases, you may need to supplement your CBE documentation by using nurses' progress notes.

*Nursing diagnoses-based standardized care plans.* You'll use these preprinted care plans whenever you identify a nursing diagnosis. Use a separate form for each pertinent diagnosis. The forms have spaces that allow you to individualize them as needed. You can, for example, include expected outcomes and major care plan revisions. Place the completed forms in the nurses' progress notes section of the clinical record.

*Nursing-medical order flow sheet.* You'll use this form to document your assessments and interventions. Each flow sheet is designed for a 24-hour period for one patient. (See *Using a nursing-medical order flow sheet.*)

The top of the form contains the orders for assessments and interventions. Each nursing order includes the corresponding nursing diagnosis number, labeled ND 1, ND 2, and so on; medical orders are identified with "DO" (doctor's orders).

After completing an assessment, compare your findings with the normal criteria defined in the printed guidelines on the back of the form. If the findings are normal, place a checkmark in the appropriate category box. If the findings aren't normal, put an asterisk in the category box. Then explain your findings in the comments section on the bottom portion of the form. Reference this note by nursing diagnosis number or doctor's order and time. If the patient's condition hasn't changed from the last assessment, draw a horizontal arrow from the previous category box to the current one.

You'll document interventions in a similar manner. Use a checkmark to indicate a completed intervention and an expected patient response. Indicate significant findings or abnormal patient responses with an asterisk, and write an explanation in the comments section. When the patient's response is unchanged, use an arrow.

After you document an entire column in the assessments and interventions section, initial it at the bottom. Also initial all your entries in the comments section, and sign the form at the bottom of the page.

*Graphic record.* You'll use this flow sheet to document trends in the patient's vital signs, weight, intake and output, stool, urine, appetite, and activity level. As with the nursing-medical order flow sheet, use checkmarks and asterisks to indicate expected and abnormal findings, respectively. Note information on abnormalities in the nurses' progress notes or on the nursing-medical order flow sheet. (See *Using a graphic record*, page 144.)

In the box labeled *routine standards*, check off that you've carried out established nursing care inter-

CHARTING

## Using a nursing-medical order flow sheet

This sample shows the typical features of a nursing-medical order flow sheet.

**NURSING-MEDICAL ORDER FLOW SHEET**

Date  1/22/92

| ND #/DO | Assessments and interventions | | | | | | | | |
|---------|-------------------------------|--|--|--|--|--|--|--|--|
| ND1 | Integumentary assessment | 1000 * | 1100 * | | | | | | |
| ND1 | Vascular assessment | 1000 ✓ | 1100 * | | | | | | |
| ND2 | Pain/comfort measure | 1000 * | 1100 → | | | | | | |
| DO | Discontinue peripheral I.V. | 1230 ✓ | | | | | | | |
| Initials | | BAL | BAL | | | | | | |

**Key**
DO = doctor's orders
ND = nursing diagnosis
✓ = normal findings

→ = no change in condition
* = abnormal or significant finding
(See Comments section.)

| ND #/DO | Time | Comments | Initials |
|---------|------|----------|----------|
| ND1 | 1000 | Ⓛ lower leg wound dressing saturated with pink-yellow nonodorous drainage. Redressed. Will reassess q1hr. ——— | |
| ND2 | 1000 | Pt. reports pain in Ⓛ lower leg at 8 on a scale of 1 to 10. Administered Percocet. | BAL |
| ND1 | 1100 | No drainage on Ⓛ lower leg dressing. | BAL |
| ND2 | 1100 | Pt. reports pain improved to a 3. | BAL |
| | | | BAL |

| INITIALS | SIGNATURE |
|----------|-----------|
| BAL | Barbara A. Lane, RN |

CHARTING

## Using a graphic record

This partial form illustrates how to use a typical graphic record.

### GRAPHIC RECORD

| Date | 1-22-92 | | | | | | 1-23-92 | | | | | | | | |
|---|---|---|---|---|---|---|---|---|---|---|---|---|---|---|---|
| Hour | 2 | 6 | 10 | 14 | 18 | 22 | 6 | 10 | 14 | | | | | | |
| Temperature | | | | | | | | | | | | | | | |

Temperature scale:
| °C | °F |
|---|---|
| 40.6° | 105° |
| 40.0° | 104° |
| 39.4° | 103° |
| 38.9° | 102° |
| 38.3° | 101° |
| 37.8° | 100° |
| 37.2° | 99° |
| 37.0° | 98.6° |
| 36.7° | 98° |
| 36.1° | 97° |
| 35.6° | 96° |

| | | | | | | | | | |
|---|---|---|---|---|---|---|---|---|---|
| Pulse | 72 | 80 | 74 | 68 | 70 | 68 | 72 | 70 | |
| Respirations | 16 | 16 | 18 | 16 | 18 | 16 | 16 | 18 | |
| BP | 6  132/86 | | 18  128/82 | | | | 6  128/82 | | |
| | 10  138/86 | | | | | | 10  128/80 | | |
| | 14  136/86 | | | | | | | | |
| Appetite | | ✓ | | ✓ | | | | | |
| Routine standards | ✓ | ✓ | | ✓ | | ✓ | ✓ | | |
| Activity 11 to 7 | Sleeping | | | | | | Sleeping | | |
| 7 to 3 | OOB x 3 without assist | | | | | | OOB as desired | | |
| 3 to 11 | OOB x2 with assist | | | | | | | | |

ventions, such as providing hygiene. Don't rewrite these standards as orders on the nursing-medical flow sheet. Refer to the guidelines on the back of the graphic record for complete instructions.

*Patient-teaching record.* Use this form to identify the knowledge and psychomotor skills that your patient or his significant other must learn by a predetermined date. The patient-teaching record includes teaching resources, dates of patient achievements, and other pertinent observations. You may use more than one form for a patient with multiple learning needs.

*Patient discharge note.* Similar to other such forms, the patient discharge note is a flow sheet for documenting ongoing discharge planning. Follow the instructions for use printed on the back of the form.

*Nurses' progress notes.* In the CBE format, you'll use the progress notes to document care plan revisions as well as interventions that don't lend themselves to the nursing-medical order flow sheet. Because the CBE format permits you to document most assessments and interventions on the nursing-medical order flow sheet, your progress notes typically won't contain much information on assessments and interventions.

**Advantages.** The CBE format has several important advantages. By including only information that deviates from the expected, it decreases the amount of documentation needed, eliminates redundant charting, and clearly identifies abnormal data. The use of well-defined protocols and standards of care promotes uniform nursing practice. Plus, the flow sheets allow you to easily track patient trends.

One more point: All flow sheets are kept at the patient's bedside, where they serve as a ready reference. This location also tends to encourage immediate documentation.

**Disadvantages.** The chief drawback of the CBE format is the major time commitment needed to develop clear protocols and standards of care. To ensure a legally sound patient record, these protocols and standards must be in place and understood by all nursing staff members before the format can be implemented. This radically different approach to documentation takes time for people to learn, accept, and use correctly.

# Documenting patient teaching

With each patient, you'll need to implement the teaching plan you've created and evaluate its effectiveness. And, of course, you need to clearly and completely document your teaching sessions and the results. Doing so provides a permanent legal record of the extent and success of teaching. Thus, your documentation may serve as your defense against charges of insufficient patient care — even years later. Your clear documentation also helps administrators gauge the overall worth of a specific patient-education program. And your documentation can help you demonstrate cost-effectiveness or support your requests for improving patient care.

### Direct benefits
Documenting exactly what you've taught the patient also saves time by preventing duplication of patient-teaching efforts by other staff members. By checking your notes, another nurse can determine precisely what's been covered and what she should teach next, without skipping essential information. This is particularly important for patients with complicated needs who may receive care from several nurses.

Take the case of a hypertensive patient who requires instruction in several areas, including diet, medication, exercise, and self-care. Successful teaching hinges on a clear record of what's been taught by everyone involved in his care. When staff members communicate by documenting what they've taught and how well the patient has learned, the teaching plan can be evaluated and revised as needed. And the patient will get the care he deserves.

You can also use your documentation to help motivate your patient. As appropriate, you can show him your record of his learning successes and encourage him to continue. Moreover, by recording the patient's response to your teaching and your assessment of his progress, you're gathering some of the data necessary to evaluate the effectiveness of your teaching, the patient's degree of knowledge or competency, and the appropriateness of his learning outcomes.

### Documentation tools

In many facilities, you'll document patient teaching on preprinted forms that become part of the clinical record. Using these forms not only makes documentation quicker, but also ensures that it's complete.

If your facility doesn't have a preprinted form, you might talk to your supervisor about developing one. In the meantime, write accurate, detailed narrative notes to document your patient teaching. (See *Patient teaching: Using narrative notes.*)

Whether you use a preprinted form or narrative notes, keep these tips in mind:

• Check your facility's policies and procedures regarding when, where, and how to document your teaching.

• Each shift, ask yourself these questions: "What part of the teaching plan did I complete?" and "What other teaching have I given this patient or his significant other?" Then document your answers.

• Be sure your documentation indicates that the patient's ongoing educational needs are being met.

• Before discharge, document the patient's remaining learning needs.

*(Text continues on page 150.)*

## Patient teaching: Using narrative notes

Although many facilities use forms for documenting patient teaching, some still use narrative notes. The narrative method takes longer, of course, but it can be just as effective and accurate. The key below lists the types of information you need to document, and the example on the next page – for a patient with Parkinson's disease – illustrates how to include that information.

1. Date and time of each teaching session
2. Patient's name and patient number on every record page
3. Patient's health status and corresponding learning needs
4. Precise learning outcomes agreed on by health care team and patient
5. Identified learning enhancements
6. Actual teaching you carry out
7. Specific teaching techniques
8. Patient's characteristics as a learner
9. Precise description of exactly what occurred, avoiding broad terms such as "learned well" and "seems to understand"
10. Your evaluation of patient's change or learning
11. Patient's response to teaching and learning experience, using his own words and behaviors
12. Specific teaching materials
13. Indications that patient or family member understands instructions
14. Identified learning barriers
15. Final progress notes with discharge teaching about diet, medications, physical activity, and follow-up care
16. Your signature

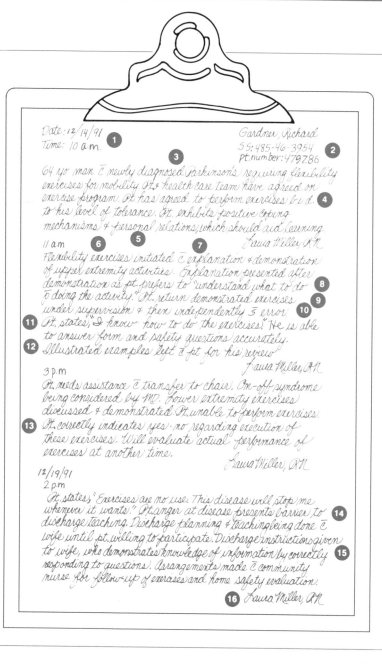

Date: 12/14/91 **(1)**                    Gardner, Richard
Time: 10 a.m.                              SS: 485-46-3954 **(2)**
                        **(3)**            Pt. number: 479286

64 y/o man c̄ newly diagnosed Parkinson's requiring flexibility
exercises for mobility. Pt. & health care team have agreed on
exercise program. Pt. has agreed to perform exercises b i d. **(4)**
to his level of tolerance. Pt. exhibits positive coping
mechanisms & personal relations, which should aid learning
11 a.m **(6)**   **(5)**          **(7)**          Laura Miller, RN

Flexibility exercises initiated c̄ explanation & demonstration
of upper extremity activities. Explanation presented after
demonstration as pt. prefers to "understand what to do **(8)**
p̄ doing the activity." Pt. return demonstrated exercises **(9)**
under supervision & then independently s̄ error. **(10)**
**(11)** Pt. states, "I know how to do the exercises." He is able
to answer form and safety questions accurately.
**(12)** Illustrated examples left c̄ pt. for his review
                                          Laura Miller, RN

3 p.m
Pt. needs assistance c̄ transfer to chair. On-off syndrome
being considered by MD. Lower extremity exercises
discussed & demonstrated. Pt. unable to perform exercises.
**(13)** Pt. correctly indicates yes-no regarding execution of
these exercises. Will evaluate actual performance of
exercises at another time.
                                          Laura Miller, RN

12/19/91
2 p.m
 Pt. states, "Exercises are no use. This disease will stop me
whenever it wants." Pt. anger at disease presents barrier to **(14)**
discharge teaching. Discharge planning & teaching being done c̄
wife until pt. willing to participate. Discharge instructions given
to wife, who demonstrates knowledge of information by correctly **(15)**
responding to questions. Arrangements made c̄ community
nurse for follow-up of exercises and home safety evaluation.
                        **(16)** Laura Miller, RN

CHARTING

## Discharge summary and patient instruction form

This sample form combines your discharge summary with your postdischarge instructions for the patient. You'd give a copy of this form to the patient at discharge.

---

### DISCHARGE SUMMARY

Date _1 / 25 / 92_
Time _2 p.m._

**Destination**
☑ Home
☐ Nursing home
☐ Other_____

**Mobility**
☑ Ambulatory
☐ Wheelchair
☐ Stretcher

**PATIENT STATUS**
General
☑ TPR _98.6° – 76 – 16_
☑ BP _134/82_
☐ Eating regularly
Comments _____

**Skin**
☑ Good condition
☑ Wound _①leg wound healing well_
☐ Other _____

**Bowels**
☐ Regular movement
☐ Irregular movement
☐ Ostomy

**Bladder**
☑ Continent
☐ Urinary frequency
☐ Incontinent
☐ Catheter
Type _____
Date changed _____

**Compliance**
☑ Understands physical condition
☑ Willing to comply with regimen
☑ States understanding of instructions
Comments _Gave successful return_
_demonstration of ① leg wound_
_dressing change._

**Medications**
☐ Preadmission medications returned
_____
☑ Prescriptions given to patient
_____
☐ Medications given to patient
_____
☑ Patient or family knows of allergies

Nurse's signature _Barbara Q. Lane, RN_

---

### PATIENT INSTRUCTIONS

**Diet**
☑ Unrestricted
☐ Restricted _____

**Activity**
☑ Walking
☑ Climbing stairs
☑ Riding in car
☑ Driving car
☑ Showering

☐ Taking a tub bath
☑ Engaging in
sexual intercourse
☑ Resuming regular
activity
☑ Lifting
☐ Exercising

☐ Other _____
Comments: _Avoid strenuous exercise_
_until wound completely heals._

**Medications**

Percocet

**Dosage, time, and route**

1 tablet orally every
6 hours as needed for
pain relief.

**Special instructions**

**Referral**

☑ Call Dr. Wilson _____ and schedule an appointment 2 weeks from today

☐ Home care agency _____

☐ Other _____

If you have questions, call Dr. Wilson _____ at 555-193

I've read and understood these instructions,
and I've received a copy of this form.

Date 1/25/92

Patient or significant other

Janice Hart

Nurse and doctor

Barbara A. Lane, RN    Dr. H. Wilson, MD

# Documenting patient discharge

JCAHO requirements specify that when preparing a patient for discharge, you must document your assessment of his continuing care needs as well as referrals for such care. To facilitate this documentation (and to save charting time), many facilities have developed combined discharge summaries and patient instructions. (See *Discharge summary and patient instruction form*, pages 148 and 149.)

This documentation tool combines all the essential information required on a discharge summary as well as the instructions given to the patient. Typically, you'll keep one copy of the form in the clinical record and give one copy to the patient. The copy you keep can then provide useful information for further teaching and evaluation.

Of course, not all facilities use these forms. Some still require a narrative discharge summary. If you must use this type of documentation, be sure to include the following information:
• patient's status on admission and discharge
• significant highlights of the hospitalization
• outcomes of your interventions
• resolved and unresolved patient problems, continuing care needs for unresolved problems, and referrals for continuing care
• instructions given to the patient or significant other about medications, treatments, activity, diet, referrals, and follow-up appointments, as well as any other special instructions.

## Suggested readings

Burke, L., and Murphy, J. *Charting by Exception: A Cost-Effective Quality Approach.* New York: John Wiley & Sons, 1988.

Cline, A. "Streamlined Documentation Through Exceptional Charting," *Nursing Management* 20(2):62-64, February 1989.

*Documentation.* Clinical Pocket Manual. Springhouse, Pa: Springhouse Corp., 1987.

Edelstein, J. "A Study of Nursing Documentation," *Nursing Management* 21(11):43, 46, November 1990.

Eggland, E.T. "Charting: How and Why to Document Your Care Daily—And Fully," *Nursing88* 18(11):76-79, 81-84, November 1988.

Iyer, P.W. "New Trends in Charting," *Nursing91* 21 (1):48-50, January 1991.

Iyer, P.W., and Camp, N.H. *Nursing Documentation: A Nursing Process Approach.* Philadelphia: Mosby Yearbook, Inc., 1991.

Lampe, S.S. "Focus Charting: Streamlining Documentation," *Nursing Management* 16(7):43-45, July 1985.

Morton, P.G. *Health Assessment in Nursing.* Springhouse, Pa.: Springhouse Corp., 1989.

*Patient-Teaching Looseleaf Library.* Springhouse, Pa.: Springhouse Corp., 1990.

# SELF-TEST

Test your documentation knowledge and skills at your own pace by answering the multiple-choice questions on pages 152 to 156. Answers appear on page 156. Then read the case history on pages 157 and 158 and fill out the initial assessment form on pages 159 to 162. A correctly completed form appears on pages 163 to 166.

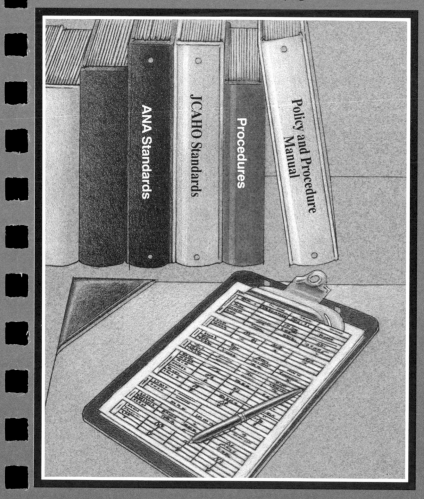

**1.** *Which forms should you use to document assessment information?*
a. the nursing care plan and the Kardex
b. the initial assessment form and flow sheets
c. the problem list and progress notes
d. protocols and graphic recordings

**2.** *In recent years, increasing emphasis has been placed on documenting:*
a. outcomes.
b. vital signs.
c. interventions.
d. patient preferences.

**3.** *Which of the following is not a quality assurance standard?*
a. structure
b. process
c. outcome
d. intervention

**4.** *If you're documenting data, action, and response, you're using:*
a. Focus charting.
b. problem-oriented charting.
c. problem-intervention-evaluation (PIE) charting.
d. charting by exception.

**5.** *Which documentation format calls for you to record only abnormal findings?*
a. Focus charting
b. charting by exception
c. PIE charting
d. narrative charting

**6.** *Which software program allows you to document nursing actions in the electronic record?*
a. nursing information system
b. computer-generated system
c. electronic nursing action system
d. nursing process system

**7.** *Peer review organizations (PROs):*
a. monitor the quality of care in health care facilities.
b. accredit health care facilities.
c. certify health care facilities for qualifying agencies.
d. research effective payment systems.

**8.** *To assess the quality of care, quality assurance monitors use well-defined, objective standards known as:*
a. processes.
b. policies.
c. indicators.
d. structures.

**9.** *The clinical record:*
a. is not admissible in court.
b. must include full signatures — never initials — for every entry.
c. always must remain at the patient's bedside.
d. verifies the quality of care provided.

**10.** *When you use a standardized care plan, you must:*
a. tailor it to fit your patient's needs.
b. plan for extra documentation time to complete it.
c. also use protocols.
d. keep in mind that it's based on the patient's signs and symptoms.

**11.** *Which documentation tool allows you to quickly compare data?*
a. flow sheet
b. protocol
c. focus sheet
d. initial assessment form

**12.** *Which documentation tool provides you with specific steps to follow for a particular nursing diagnosis?*
a. Kardex
b. protocol
c. traditional care plan
d. PIE charting

**13.** *The standards of the American Nurses' Association (ANA) require that you:*
a. base your documentation on a nursing model.
b. use flow sheets to document your assessments.
c. provide continuous documentation that's accessible to all members of the health care team.
d. make sure your documentation reflects your best medical judgment.

**14.** *If you're ever a defendant in a malpractice suit, your actions will be compared with:*
a. those of the attending doctor.
b. the expected actions of a nurse in a similar situation as defined by national standards.
c. those of a nurse manager.
d. the patient's expectations.

**15.** *If you make a mistake in the clinical record, you should:*
a. white it out, then sign and date it.
b. completely cross it out using ink.
c. draw a single line through it, write "mistaken entry" above or beside it, and initial and date your correction.
d. erase it completely, write in the correct information, and initial and date the entry.

**16.** *Which of the following will a court accept as evidence of a patient's care?*
a. the sworn statement of the doctor
b. the sworn statement of the patient
c. the sworn statement of the nurse
d. the clinical record

**17.** *Federal Medicare regulations do:*
a. not have the authority of statutory law.
b. not influence federal reimbursement procedures.
c. not stipulate documentation requirements.
d. require health care facilities to periodically update the requirements for participation in Medicare.

**18.** *For a health care facility to receive accreditation, the Joint Commission on Accreditation of Healthcare Organizations (JCAHO) requires:*
a. documentation of patient self-care capabilities.
b. the use of traditional nursing care plans.
c. the use of nursing diagnoses.
d. the inclusion of incident reports in the clinical record.

**19.** *Your legal signature on the clinical record should include your:*
a. first initial, full last name, and professional licensure.
b. full first name, middle initial, full last name, and licensure.

c. full legal name, licensure, and academic credentials.
d. last name, followed by a comma and your full first name, academic credentials, and licensure.

**20.** *You may legally countersign a document to:*
a. indicate your overall responsibility for an LPN under your supervision.
b. show you understand the orders of another health care professional, such as a physical therapist.
c. verify that you've transcribed a doctor's orders to the correct forms.
d. verify another nurse's accuracy.

**21.** *What do state and provincial laws on documentation have in common?*
a. Neither mandates health care facilities to document.
b. Both provide the same regulations for documentation.
c. Both require documentation of clinical practice in health care facilities, although specific laws vary.
d. Both provide the most stringent legal requirements for clinical documentation.

**22.** *ANA standards carry so much weight because they:*
a. have the binding power of statutory law.
b. affect both LPNs and RNs.
c. represent a national consensus.
d. are formulated in conjunction with the National League for Nursing.

**23.** *Informed consent requires all of the following* except:
a. a description of the risks the treatment poses.
b. an explanation of the consequences of refusing treatment.
c. confirmation that the patient is legally competent to give informed consent.
d. an explanation that consent can't be withdrawn once it's been given.

**24.** *When can you legally perform a procedure against the wishes of a competent patient?*
a. never
b. when two competent, immediate family members request the procedure

c. when the health care facility or doctor obtains a court order
d. when a doctor who's willing to take full responsibility gives you an order

**25.** *When a patient leaves the hospital against medical advice (AMA), the discharge form should* not *say that he:*
a. understands that he's leaving AMA.
b. has been advised of, understands, and accepts the risks of leaving.
c. knows he can return to the hospital.
d. understands that he should go to another health care facility for future treatment.

**26.** *The main purpose of an incident report is to:*
a. inform administrators that an incident occurred so they can take steps to prevent a recurrence.
b. serve as proof that the incident took place.
c. name those responsible for the incident.
d. prevent a liability claim.

**27.** *Who should sign an incident report?*
a. only the nurse supervisor
b. only someone with first-hand knowledge of the incident
c. only a doctor
d. only a reliable patient

**28.** *An incident report should include:*
a. your conclusions about the cause of the incident.
b. suggestions for preventing a recurrence of the incident.
c. opinions about the nature of the incident from other health care workers.
d. a description of the incident and its consequences to the patient.

**29.** *When you complete an incident report, make sure you:*
a. file it in the patient's clinical record.
b. note in the clinical record that you filed an incident report.
c. consult a lawyer.
d. include details about the incident in your progress notes.

**30.** *Which of the following statements is true?*

a. As long as you follow a nursing care plan, you don't have to document assessment information.
b. You should complete your assessment at the initial interview.
c. Your documented assessment data is admissible as evidence in a court of law.
d. You should include only the assessment information you obtain from the patient.

**31.** *Which of the following determines how long a health care facility allows for initial assessments?*
a. the acuity level of the patient population being assessed
b. the facility's need to establish a uniform time limit for all initial assessments
c. the number of patients who need an initial assessment
d. the average length of hospitalization at the facility

**32.** *You obtain subjective information by:*
a. observing your patient.
b. performing a physical examination.
c. checking laboratory reports.
d. listening to your patient's descriptions of his symptoms.

**33.** *Primary sources of assessment information include:*
a. the patient's family.
b. the patient.
c. the patient's previous clinical records.
d. other members of the health care team.

**34.** *Which of the following statements best describes general observations?*
a. They provide critical clues about patient problems.
b. They lead you to draw conclusions from your initial impressions.
c. They yield minimal information.
d. They take a long time to complete.

**35.** *You'll collect a health history for all of the following reasons* except:
a. to assess the impact of an illness on the patient and his family.
b. to determine the patient's learning needs.
c. to initiate discharge planning.
d. to plan medical treatment.

**36.** *You must include discharge planning, the patient's self-care capabilities and learning needs, and biophysical, psycho-social, and environmental factors in your initial assessment because:*
a. these are integral parts of the health history.
b. they provide a complete picture of the patient.
c. the JCAHO requires them.
d. PROs require them.

**37.** *Which method allows you to document your initial assessment most completely and efficiently?*
a. narrative notes
b. a standardized, open-ended method
c. a standardized, close-ended method
d. whichever method meets the needs of the particular patient

**38.** *The North American Nursing Diagnosis Association bases its classification system for nursing diagnoses on:*
a. the medical model.
b. human response patterns.
c. functional health care patterns.
d. the patient's ability to function independently.

**39.** *Taken together, a human response or problem, related factors, and signs and symptoms make up:*
a. a nursing diagnosis.
b. a medical diagnosis.
c. the case management system.
d. the initial assessment.

**40.** *What does the related-to statement in a nursing diagnosis help you determine?*
a. patient outcomes
b. evaluations
c. interventions
d. signs and symptoms

**41.** *Which of the following is the best outcome statement?*
a. Increases fluids
b. Understands the need to take deep breaths
c. States relief of chest pain within 1 hour of receiving medication
d. Significantly improves ability to ambulate

**42.** *What's the major drawback of the standardized care plan?*
a. It has to be tailored to fit the patient.
b. It takes time to complete.
c. It's difficult to keep current.
d. It's not as effective as a traditional care plan.

**43.** *Which of the following would be a cognitive outcome?*
a. Demonstrates how to read a thermometer correctly.
b. Complies with prescribed diet.
c. States the purpose of each medication.
d. Understands the disease process.

**44.** *You should begin discharge planning:*
a. before or on the day of admission.
b. several days after admission.
c. at discharge.
d. several days before discharge.

**45.** *Since the advent of diagnosis-related groups, Medicare pays:*
a. retrospectively for care provided.
b. prospectively based on the patient's diagnosis.
c. a percentage of the patient's costs, as a private insurance company would.
d. on a sliding scale based on the patient's income.

**46.** *A case management plan is:*
a. a care plan determined by the doctor.
b. a type of computerized nursing care plan.
c. a standardized time line that spells out all the events that will probably occur for a patient with a particular diagnosis.
d. a plan that focuses only on the financial outcomes of patient care.

**47.** *Which of the following is an interdependent intervention?*
a. teaching a patient to care for himself
b. taking steps to make a patient more comfortable
c. inserting an indwelling urinary catheter
d. turning a patient every 2 hours

**48.** *Narrative charting:*
a. encourages you to follow the nursing process in documentation.
b. helps you to write clear, organized nursing notes.

c. provides a forum for health care team members to communicate.
d. meets JCAHO documentation requirements.

**49.** *Unlike narrative and problem-oriented charting, Focus charting is designed to:*
a. save time.
b. help you write clear nursing notes.
c. encourage you to follow the nursing process.
d. meet JCAHO requirements.

**50.** *Which charting format uses the SOAPIE method?*
a. problem-oriented
b. Focus
c. PIE
d. charting by exception

**51.** *In the SOAP charting method, you'd include a patient's complaint about a leaking dressing under:*
a. S.
b. O.
c. A.
d. P.

**52.** *In the PIE charting format, where would you include the statement, "Admin-*

*istered Demerol and assisted with repositioning from back to left side"?*
a. P
b. I
c. E
d. You wouldn't include this statement in PIE charting.

**53.** *Unlike some other charting formats, charting by exception always calls for you to use:*
a. protocols.
b. flow sheets.
c. a nursing care plan.
d. a problem list.

**54.** *Which learning outcome provides you with the most complete information?* ·
a. Recognizes unusual chest pain.
b. Understands preoperative instructions.
c. Changes eating habits.
d. States three signs of infection.

**55.** *You'll base your teaching content and methods on the patient's:*
a. physical needs.
b. psychosocial needs.
c. learning needs.
d. condition.

---

### ANSWERS

| | | | | | |
|---|---|---|---|---|---|
| **1.** b | **11.** a | **20.** c | **29.** d | **38.** b | **47.** c |
| **2.** a | **12.** b | **21.** c | **30.** c | **39.** a | **48.** d |
| **3.** d | **13.** c | **22.** c | **31.** a | **40.** c | **49.** a |
| **4.** a | **14.** b | **23.** d | **32.** d | **41.** c | **50.** a |
| **5.** b | **15.** c | **24.** c | **33.** b | **42.** a | **51.** a |
| **6.** a | **16.** d | **25.** d | **34.** a | **43.** c | **52.** b |
| **7.** a | **17.** a | **26.** a | **35.** d | **44.** a | **53.** a |
| **8.** c | **18.** a | **27.** b | **36.** c | **45.** b | **54.** d |
| **9.** d | **19.** a | **28.** d | **37.** d | **46.** c | **55.** c |
| **10.** a | | | | | |

Read the case history below and use the information to complete the initial assessment form beginning on page 159. Then check your documentation against the properly completed form starting on page 163.

At 2 p.m. on December 10, 1991, Jane Stephanowicz, a 54-year-old marketing manager, is admitted with a diagnosis of dysfunctional uterine bleeding and assigned to room 226A. Her doctor, Harold Samuelson, has scheduled her for a total hysterectomy early the next morning.

*Initial interview and observations.* As you talk with Mrs. Stephanowicz and orient her to the room, you find that she's alert and articulate. She tells you that she's a college graduate and enjoys skiing and crafts. Her husband is a salesman and they have an adopted son, age 20. She also mentions that she's a practicing Roman Catholic. When questioned, she explains that she would like to receive the Sacrament of the Sick before surgery.

Mrs. Stephanowicz states that she has come to the hospital "to have a hysterectomy because of uterine bleeding." She understands and describes her problem and its treatment very well. She says she's "somewhat anxious" about the surgery. Later she admits that she's really more afraid of the postoperative pain than she is of the procedure itself. What's more, she thinks about this "all the time" and, as a result, has slept poorly for the past three nights.

Mrs. Stephanowicz also says that her marketing job is very demanding and that she's worried her recovery will take longer than the 3 weeks she's planned for. She fears that a longer recovery would require her to take a leave of absence, but she can't afford the loss of income. She says her husband has been very supportive and that he'll be able to assist her in any way when she's discharged from the hospital. As she states her concerns, you note that she constantly shifts in her chair.

*Exploring the chief complaint.* Mrs. Stephanowicz tells you that she's had irregular uterine bleeding for over a year and that recently it has gotten worse and become painful. The pain, she tells you, "comes and goes" in her lower abdomen and feels like an ache. She also says that she has been tiring quickly and "has a general lack of ambition." As you explore the problem further, you learn that Mrs. Stephanowicz underwent a dilatation and curettage in February 1991. She tells you that this procedure seemed to solve the problem for about 3 months, when the bleeding started again.

*Collecting related history data.* Mrs. Stephanowicz can't remember when her menarche occurred. Her last menstrual period was "about 2½ years ago." She's had a Pap test annually and had her last one in November 1990. She says she has no chest pain or leg pain. She also has no pain on breathing and doesn't use any type of adjunctive oxygen at home.

Mrs. Stephanowicz says that she occasionally has a problem with constipation, for which she takes Senokot. She hasn't had any constipation in the past month. Her last bowel movement was yesterday afternoon. The constipation is her only problem related to bowel movements; she has no history of urinary problems.

She states further that she is allergic to penicillin but is not now taking any medications. She's never smoked. She enjoys a glass of wine on special occasions but otherwise does not drink alcoholic beverages. She also tells you that she has no history of seizures or dizziness, and she has never walked in her sleep.

Mrs. Stephanowicz states that her weight has been constant over the past 5 years. She tells you that she has no food intolerances but has noticed occasional heartburn after eating spicy foods. She says she has a good appetite. She also tells you that she has no chewing or swallowing difficulty and that she hasn't experienced nausea or vomiting recently. She wears glasses for reading and says she has no difficulty hearing.

***General appearance.*** A stocky woman, Mrs. Stephanowicz weighs 160 lb and is 5′ 5″ tall. Her hair is light brown with streaks of gray. She walks well without assistance, and her gait is normal. Her body movements are smooth, symmetrical, and coordinated.

Her whitish pink skin has a normal texture and gives off no noticeable odor. She has two light brown, rounded nevi (one on the left lower abdominal quadrant about 2.5 mm in diameter, and the other on the upper right arm about 2 mm in diameter). She has one scar about 6 cm long on the right lower abdominal quadrant that she says resulted from an appendectomy at age 9.

Her teeth are normal; she has several fillings but no obvious untreated caries. The gums and tongue are pink and moist. Her breath odor is unremarkable.

***Vital signs.*** Mrs. Stephanowicz's vital signs are: temperature, 98.6° F (37° C); radial pulse rate, 86 beats/minute; respiratory rate, 16 breaths/minute; and blood pressure, 118/80 (right arm) and 120/82 (left arm). Her heart sounds are normal, with no audible murmurs. The apical heart rate is 86 beats/minute. All pulses have a regular rhythm and a normal rate. The extremity temperatures are normal. Extremity pulses are palpable with a regular rate and rhythm. Capillary filling is adequate. Her respiratory rate and rhythm are regular, and lung sounds are normal. You don't note any shortness of breath or coughing.

***GI and genitourinary findings.*** As you auscultate bowel sounds, you note no abdominal distention. Mrs. Stephanowicz doesn't have an ostomy. A rectal examination reveals two small external hemorrhoids but no rectal bleeding.

***Personal possessions.*** During her hospital stay, Mrs. Stephanowicz will keep two knee-length nightgowns — one with a pink-flower print, the other plain yellow; a white floor-length robe; and a pair of white terry-cloth slippers. She'll also keep one yellow metal ladies' watch, a plain white gold wedding band, five $1 bills and 75¢ in change, and her yellow wire-rimmed reading glasses.

**BLANK INITIAL ASSESSMENT FORM**

### INITIAL ASSESSMENT

#### GENERAL INFORMATION

Age___ Sex___ Height___ Weight_____

T___ P___ R___ B/P(R)___ (L)_____

Room_____ Admission time_____
Admission date_____
Doctor_____
Admitting diagnosis_____

Patient's stated reason for
hospitalization _____

**Medical history**

**Allergies**
_____
_____
_____

**Current medications**

| Name | Dosage | Last taken |
|---|---|---|
|  |  |  |
|  |  |  |

**Orientation**
☐ Identification band
☐ Visiting policy
☐ Smoking policy
☐ Bed position and side rails
☐ Call light
☐ Intercom

☐ Television
☐ Telephone
☐ Bathroom
☐ Signed consent

I understand the explanations I've received during orientation.
Patient's signature_____

**Personal possessions**
☐ Money _____
☐ Clothing _____
_____
_____
☐ Jewelry _____

☐ Glasses _____
☐ Contact lenses _____
☐ Dentures _____
☐ Hearing aid _____
☐ Other _____

#### VALUING

Religion _____
_____

☐ Request for clerical visit
☐ Request for religious rites_____

#### SUBJECTIVE DATA

☐ From patient   ☐ From other

#### OBJECTIVE DATA

#### RELATING, CHOOSING

☐ Single    ☐ Divorced
☐ Married   ☐ Widowed
Most supportive person _____
☐ Alcohol use
How much_____  How often_____
☐ Substance abuse
Type_____

Pertinent nonverbal behavior _____
_____

Describe patient's ability to comply with
therapy for long-term health problems.
_____
_____
_____

Date_____ Signature_____

*(continued)*

## INITIAL ASSESSMENT

| SUBJECTIVE DATA | OBJECTIVE DATA |
|---|---|

☐ From patient    ☐ From other

### EXCHANGING

**Oxygenation**

Yes   No
☐    ☐ Dyspnea _____
☐    ☐ Painful breathing _____
☐    ☐ Cough _____
☐    ☐ Sputum _____
☐    ☐ Use of oxygen at home _____
Smoking history _____

☐ Regular respirations
☐ Irregular respirations _____
☐ Normal breath sounds
☐ Abnormal breath sounds _____
_____

**Circulation**

Yes   No
☐    ☐ Chest pain _____
☐    ☐ Palpitations _____
☐    ☐ Leg pain _____
☐    ☐ Limbs numb _____
☐    ☐ Limbs cold _____

☐ Regular heart rhythm
☐ Irregular heart rhythm _____
☐ Normal heart sounds
☐ Abnormal heart sounds _____
☐ Adequate capillary refill _____
☐ Edema _____
Apical rate _____ Radial rate _____
Carotid pulse R ___ Radial pulse R _____
Femoral pulse R ___ Pedal pulse R _____
Comments _____

**Reproduction**

☐ Menarche
Last menstrual period _____
Last Pap smear _____

**Tissue, skin integrity**

Yes   No
☐    ☐ Dry _____
☐    ☐ Pale _____
☐    ☐ Itchy _____
☐    ☐ Bruised _____
☐    ☐ Other _____
_____
_____

☐ Flushed
☐ Pale
☐ Cyanotic
☐ Pink
☐ Dry
☐ Moist
☐ Cool
☐ Warm

Mark illustrations, using key.
1 Blister _____ 6 Rash _____
2 Bruise _____ 7 Scar _____
3 Burn _____ 8 Ulcer _____
4 Pressure ulcer ___ 9 Wound _____
5 Nevi _____ 10 Other _____
_____

Date_____ Signature_____

**INITIAL ASSESSMENT**                                                          page 3

| SUBJECTIVE DATA | OBJECTIVE DATA |
|---|---|

☐ From patient      ☐ From other

## NUTRITION

Yes  No
☐    ☐  Recent weight gain
☐    ☐  Recent weight loss
☐    ☐  Recent increase in appetite
☐    ☐  Recent decrease in appetite
☐    ☐  Food intolerance
☐    ☐  Nausea
☐    ☐  Vomiting
☐    ☐  Heartburn
☐    ☐  Swallowing problems
Diet _____
Comments _____
_____
_____
_____

Breath:            Teeth:           Gums:
☐ Normal           ☐ Normal         ☐ Moist
☐ Fruity           ☐ Caries         ☐ Pink
☐ Halitosis        ☐ Loose          ☐ Pale
☐ Other _____    ☐ Broken         ☐ Bleeding
                   ☐ Missing ___

Tongue:            Body type:
☐ Moist            ☐ Normal
☐ Dry              ☐ Thin
☐ Pink             ☐ Emaciated
☐ Other _____    ☐ Obese

### Elimination
Yes  No
☐    ☐  Continent (urine)
☐    ☐  Continent (stool)
☐    ☐  Urinary problems _____
☐    ☐  Constipation
☐    ☐  Hemorrhoids _____
☐    ☐  Rectal bleeding _____
Date of last bowel movement _____
Patient's constipation remedy _____

☐ Bowel sounds
☐ Abdominal distention
☐ Ostomy _____
☐ Urinary catheter _____
   Appearance of urine _____
   Appearance of diarrheic stool _____
   Comments _____

## MOVING

### Rest, activity, self-care
Yes  No
☐    ☐  Ambulates _____
☐    ☐  Bathes self _____
☐    ☐  Paralysis _____
☐    ☐  Seizures _____
☐    ☐  Sleeping problems _____
_____
_____
Activities _____

☐ Steady gait
☐ Unsteady gait
☐ Cane
☐ Walker
☐ Moves limbs _____
☐ Has stiffness _____
☐ Contractures _____
☐ Deformities _____
☐ Amputation _____

Date_____ Signature_____

*(continued)*

## INITIAL ASSESSMENT

### SUBJECTIVE DATA

☐ From patient    ☐ From other

### OBJECTIVE DATA

### PERCEIVING, COMMUNICATING

Yes    No

☐       ☐ Visual impairment _____

        _____

☐       ☐ Hearing impairment _____

☐ Other sensory impairment _____

_____

_____

☐ Alert
☐ Lethargic
☐ Semicomatose
☐ Unconscious

☐ Ocular drainage _____
☐ Ear drainage _____
☐ Normal speech
☐ Abnormal speech _____
☐ Language barrier _____

### FEELING

Yes    No

☐       ☐ Pain not noted elsewhere _____

        _____

☐       ☐ Recent loss _____

☐ Calm
☐ Apprehensive
☐ Grimaces _____
☐ Guarding _____
☐ Other signs of pain _____

_____

### KNOWING

Highest grade completed _____
☐ Reads English
☐ Reads other language _____
☐ Understanding of illness _____

_____

_____

_____

☐ Answers questions appropriately
☐ Follows directions
☐ Teaching needs _____

_____

_____

_____

### DISCHARGE PLANNING

Patient and family postdischarge intentions

_____

_____

_____

_____

_____

Date_____ Signature_____

**COMPLETED INITIAL ASSESSMENT FORM**

### INITIAL ASSESSMENT

#### GENERAL INFORMATION

Age 54 Sex F Height 5'5" Weight 160 lbs

T 98.6 P 86 R 16 B/P(R) 118/80 (L) 120/82

Room 226 A   Admission time 2 p.m.
Admission date 12/10/91
Doctor H. Samuelson

Admitting diagnosis Dysfunctional uterine bleeding

Patient's stated reason for hospitalization "to have a hysterectomy because of uterine bleeding."

**Medical history**
Appendectomy, age 9

**Orientation**
- ☑ Identification band
- ☑ Visiting policy
- ☑ Smoking policy
- ☑ Bed position and side rails
- ☑ Call light
- ☑ Intercom
- ☑ Television
- ☑ Telephone
- ☑ Bathroom
- ☑ Signed consent

I understand the explanations I've received during orientation.
Patient's signature Jane Stephanowicz

**Personal possessions**
- ☑ Money $5.75
- ☑ Clothing two knee-length nightgowns (pink flowered and yellow), white robe, one pair white terry-cloth slippers.
- ☑ Jewelry yellow metal ladies' watch, one white gold wedding band.
- ☑ Glasses yellow wire-rimmed reading glasses
- ☐ Contact lenses
- ☐ Dentures
- ☐ Hearing aid
- ☐ Other

**Allergies**
Penicillin

**Current medications**

| Name | Dosage | Last taken |
|------|--------|------------|
| None |        |            |
|      |        |            |
|      |        |            |

#### VALUING

Religion Roman Catholic

- ☑ Request for clerical visit
- ☑ Request for religious rites Sacrament of Sick before surgery

#### SUBJECTIVE DATA

☑ From patient    ☐ From other

#### OBJECTIVE DATA

#### RELATING, CHOOSING

- ☐ Single        ☐ Divorced
- ☑ Married       ☐ Widowed

Most supportive person Husband
- ☑ Alcohol use
How much 1 glass of wine How often Special occasions
- ☐ Substance abuse
Type none

Pertinent nonverbal behavior Constantly changes position in chair

Describe patient's ability to comply with therapy for long-term health problems.
NA

Date 12/10/91   Signature J. Celena, RN

*(continued)*

INITIAL ASSESSMENT                                          page 2

| **SUBJECTIVE DATA** | **OBJECTIVE DATA** |
|---|---|

☑ From patient   ☐ From other

**EXCHANGING**

**Oxygenation**

Yes   No
☐     ☑ Dyspnea _____        ☑ Regular respirations
☐     ☑ Painful breathing _____   ☐ Irregular respirations _____
☐     ☑ Cough _____       ☑ Normal breath sounds
☐     ☑ Sputum _____      ☐ Abnormal breath sounds _____
☐     ☑ Use of oxygen at home _____
Smoking history **Never smoked**

**Circulation**

Yes   No
☐     ☑ Chest pain _____      ☑ Regular heart rhythm
☐     ☑ Palpitations _____       ☐ Irregular heart rhythm _____
☐     ☑ Leg pain _____         ☑ Normal heart sounds
☐     ☑ Limbs numb _____        ☐ Abnormal heart sounds _____
☐     ☑ Limbs cold _____       ☑ Adequate capillary refill _____
                                     ☐ Edema _____
                                     Apical rate **86** __ Radial rate **86**
                                     Carotid pulse R __ Radial pulse R ____
                                     Femoral pulse R __ Pedal pulse R ____

**Reproduction**                    Comments **All pulses palpable**
☑ Menarche
Last menstrual period **about 2½ years ago**
Last Pap smear **Nov. 1990**

**Tissue, skin integrity**

Yes   No
☐     ☑ Dry _____          ☐ Flushed
☐     ☑ Pale _____         ☐ Pale
☐     ☑ Itchy _____         ☐ Cyanotic
☐     ☑ Bruised _____          ☑ Pink
☐     ☐ Other _____          ☑ Dry
                                     ☐ Moist
                                     ☐ Cool
                                     ☐ Warm

Mark illustrations, using key.
1 Blister _____    6 Rash _____
2 Bruise _____    7 Scar **Appendectomy 6 cm**
3 Burn _____      8 Ulcer _____
4 Pressure ulcer ___   9 Wound _____
5 Nevi **LLQ 2.5mm** 10 Other _____
     **Upper ℝ arm 2mm**

Date **12/10/91** Signature **J. Celena, RN**

## INITIAL ASSESSMENT                                         page 3

| SUBJECTIVE DATA | OBJECTIVE DATA |
|---|---|

☑ From patient    ☐ From other

### NUTRITION

| Yes | No | | Breath: | Teeth: | Gums: |
|---|---|---|---|---|---|
| ☐ | ☑ | Recent weight gain | ☑ Normal | ☑ Normal | ☑ Moist |
| ☐ | ☑ | Recent weight loss | ☐ Fruity | ☐ Caries | ☑ Pink |
| ☐ | ☑ | Recent increase in appetite | ☐ Halitosis | ☐ Loose | ☐ Pale |
| ☐ | ☑ | Recent decrease in appetite | ☐ Other ___ | ☐ Broken | ☐ Bleeding |
| ☐ | ☑ | Food intolerance | | ☐ Missing ___ | |
| ☐ | ☑ | Nausea | | | |
| ☐ | ☑ | Vomiting | Tongue: | Body type: | |
| ☑ | ☐ | Heartburn | ☑ Moist | ☐ Normal | |
| ☐ | ☑ | Swallowing problems | ☐ Dry | ☐ Thin | |

Diet _____

☑ Pink    ☐ Emaciated

Comments "_occasional heartburn after_    ☐ Other ___ ☑ Obese
_eating spicy foods_"

### Elimination

| Yes | No | | |
|---|---|---|---|
| ☑ | ☐ | Continent (urine) | ☑ Bowel sounds |
| ☑ | ☐ | Continent (stool) | ☐ Abdominal distention |
| ☐ | ☑ | Urinary problems ___ | ☐ Ostomy ___ |
| ☑ | ☐ | Constipation "_occasionally_" | ☐ Urinary catheter ___ |
| ☑ | ☐ | Hemorrhoids _2 small external_ |    Appearance of urine ___ |
| ☐ | ☑ | Rectal bleeding ___ |    Appearance of diarrheic stool ___ |

Date of last bowel movement _12/9/91_       Comments ___

Patient's constipation remedy _Senokot_

### MOVING

#### Rest, activity, self-care

| Yes | No | | |
|---|---|---|---|
| ☑ | ☐ | Ambulates ___ | ☑ Steady gait |
| ☑ | ☐ | Bathes self ___ | ☐ Unsteady gait |
| ☐ | ☑ | Paralysis ___ | ☐ Cane |
| ☐ | ☑ | Seizures ___ | ☐ Walker |
| ☑ | ☐ | Sleeping problems _Has had_ | ☑ Moves limbs _without difficulty_ |

_trouble sleeping past three nights_    ☐ Has stiffness ___
☐ Contractures ___
Activities _Skiing, crafts_    ☐ Deformities ___
☐ Amputation ___

Date_12/10/91_ Signature_J. Celena, RN_

*(continued)*

---

**INITIAL ASSESSMENT** page 4

### SUBJECTIVE DATA   OBJECTIVE DATA

☑ From patient   ☐ From other

### PERCEIVING, COMMUNICATING

Yes No
☑ ☐ Visual impairment _uses_
_glasses for reading_
☐ ☑ Hearing impairment _____
☐ Other sensory impairment _____
_____
_____

☑ Alert
☐ Lethargic
☐ Semicomatose
☐ Unconscious

☐ Ocular drainage _____
☐ Ear drainage _____
☑ Normal speech
☐ Abnormal speech _____
☐ Language barrier _____

### FEELING

Yes No
☑ ☐ Pain not noted elsewhere _an_
_ache "comes and goes" in_
_lower abdomen_
☐ ☑ Recent loss _____

☐ Calm
☑ Apprehensive
☐ Grimaces _____
☐ Guarding _____
☐ Other signs of pain _____

### KNOWING

Highest grade completed _16_
☑ Reads English
☐ Reads other language _____
☑ Understanding of illness _Able to_
_accurately state problem_
_and treatments_

☑ Answers questions appropriately
☑ Follows directions
☑ Teaching needs _care required_
_after surgery including_
_activity limitations_

### DISCHARGE PLANNING

Patient and family postdischarge intentions
_Patient is planning for her husband to help her at_
_home. She feels this is all that will be necessary._

Date _12/10/91_ Signature _J. Celena, RN_

# APPENDICES
# AND
# INDEX

# COMMON ABBREVIATIONS ON DOCUMENTATION FORMS

The list below spells out the abbreviations you'll find on sample documentation forms in this book.

| | | | |
|---|---|---|---|
| **ABG** | arterial blood gas | **OOB** | out of bed |
| **ADL** | activities of daily living | **OR** | operating room |
| **BRP** | bathroom privileges | **PaCO$_2$** | partial pressure of carbon dioxide in arterial blood |
| **CCU** | coronary care unit | | |
| **CPR** | cardiopulmonary resuscitation | **PaO$_2$** | partial pressure of oxygen in arterial blood |
| **ED** | emergency department | **P.O.** | by mouth |
| **ET** | endotracheal | **p.r.n.** | as needed |
| **HCO$_3$** | bicarbonate | **PT** | physiotherapy |
| **I & O** | intake and output | **R** | right |
| **L** | left | **ROM** | range of motion |
| **LOC** | level of consciousness | **SICU** | surgical intensive care unit |
| **MICU** | medical intensive care unit | | |
| | | **Sv̄o$_2$** | mixed venous oxygen saturation |
| **NG** | nasogastric | **TPR** | temperature, pulse, respirations |
| **NPO** | nothing by mouth | | |
| **O$_2$** | oxygen | **VF** | ventricular fibrillation |

# J.C.A.H.O. DOCUMENTATION STANDARDS

In 1991, new nursing care standards established by the Joint Commission on Accreditation of Healthcare Organizations (JCAHO) went into effect. Below you'll find the standards that apply to documentation.

## STANDARD 1

Patients receive nursing care based on a documented assessment of their needs.

### Required characteristics

**1.1** Each patient's need for nursing care related to his admission is assessed by a registered nurse.

**1.1.1** The assessment is conducted either at the time of admission or within a time frame preceding or following admission that is specified in hospital policy.

**1.1.2** Aspects of data collection may be delegated by the registered nurse.

**1.1.3** Needs are reassessed when warranted by the patient's condition.

**1.2** Each patient's assessment includes consideration of biophysical, psychosocial, environmental, self-care, educational, and discharge planning factors.

**1.2.1** When appropriate, data from the patient's significant others are included in the assessment.

**1.3** Each patient's nursing care is based on identified nursing diagnoses or patient care needs and patient care standards and is consistent with the therapies of other disciplines.

**1.3.1** The patient and significant others are involved in the patient's care, as appropriate.

**1.3.2** Nursing staff members collaborate, as appropriate, with doctors and other clinical disciplines in making decisions regarding each patient's need for nursing care.

**1.3.3** Throughout the patient's stay, the patient and, as appropriate, his significant others receive education specific to the patient's health care needs.

**1.3.3.1** In preparation for discharge, continuing care needs are assessed and referrals for such care are documented in the patient's clinical record.

**1.3.4** The patient's clinical record includes documentation of:

**1.3.4.1** the initial assessments and reassessments

**1.3.4.2** the nursing diagnoses and patient care needs

**1.3.4.3** the interventions identified to meet the patient's nursing care needs

**1.3.4.4** the nursing care provided

**1.3.4.5** the patient's response to and the outcome of the care provided

**1.3.4.6** the abilities of the patient and significant others to manage continuing care needs after discharge

**1.3.5** Nursing care data related to patient assessments, the nursing care planned, nursing interventions, and patient outcomes are permanently integrated into the clinical information system (for example, the clinical record).

**1.3.5.1** Nursing care data can be identified and retrieved from the clinical information system.

## STANDARD 5

The nurse executive and other nursing leaders participate with leaders from the governing body, management, medical staff, and clinical areas in the hospital's decision-making structures and processes.

### Required characteristics

**5.5** The nurse executive, or a designee, participates in evaluating, selecting, and integrating health care technology and information management systems that support patient care needs and the efficient utilization of nursing resources.

**5.5.1** The use of efficient interactive information management systems for nursing, other clinical (for example, dietary, pharmacy, physical therapy), and nonclinical information is facilitated wherever appropriate.

# A.N.A.'S STANDARDS OF NURSING PRACTICE

The American Nurses' Association (ANA) developed the following standards of nursing practice to provide guidelines for determining quality nursing care. These standards are based on the steps of the nursing process – assessment, nursing diagnosis, planning, implementation, and evaluation. A rationale follows each standard, along with the assessment factors to use to determine if the standard has been met.

## Standard I

Collection of data about the health status of the patient is systematic and continuous. Data are accessible, communicated, and recorded.

### Rationale

Comprehensive care requires complete and ongoing collection of data to determine the patient's nursing care needs. All health status data about the patient must be available for all members of the health care team.

### Assessment factors

Health status data include:
- growth and development
- biophysical status
- emotional status
- cultural, religious, socioeconomic background
- performance of activities of daily living
- patterns of coping
- interaction patterns
- patient's perception of and satisfaction with his health status
- patient's health goals
- environment (physical, social, emotional, ecologic)
- available and accessible human and material resources.

Data are collected from:
- patient, family, friends
- health care personnel
- individuals within the immediate environment, the community, or both.

Data are obtained by:
- interview
- examination
- observation

- reading records, reports, and other materials.

The format for data collection:
- provides for a systematic collection of data
- facilitates the completeness of data collection.

Continuous collection of data is evidenced by:
- frequent updating
- recording of health status changes.

The data are:
- accessible on the patient records
- retrievable from the record-keeping systems
- confidential when appropriate.

## Standard II

Nursing diagnoses are derived from the health status data.

### Rationale

The patient's health status is the basis for determining nursing care needs. Data are analyzed and compared with norms when possible.

### Assessment factors

The patient's health status is compared with the norm to determine if there is a deviation from the norm and the degree and direction of deviation.

The patient's capabilities and limitations are identified.

Nursing diagnoses are related to and congruent with diagnoses of other professionals caring for the patient.

## Standard III

The plan of care includes goals derived from the nursing diagnoses.

### Rationale
Determining the results to be achieved is an essential part of planning care.

### Assessment factors
Goals are mutually set with the patient and other pertinent individuals:
• They are congruent with other planned therapies.
• They are stated in realistic and measurable terms.
• They are assigned a time period for achievement.
  Goals are established to maximize the patient's functional capabilities and are congruent with:
• growth and development
• biophysical status
• behavioral patterns
• human and material resources.

### Standard IV

The plan of nursing care includes priorities and the prescribed nursing measures to achieve goals derived from the nursing diagnoses.

### Rationale
Nursing actions are planned to promote, maintain, and restore the patient's well-being.

### Assessment factors
Physiologic measures are planned to prevent or control specific patient problems and are related to the nursing diagnoses and goals of care.
  Psychosocial interventions are specific to the patient's nursing care problem and to the nursing care goals.
  Teaching and learning principles are incorporated into the plan of care, and learning objectives are stated in behavioral terms.
  Approaches are planned to provide for a therapeutic environment:
• Physical environmental factors are used to influence the therapeutic environment (for example, control of noise and temperature).
• Psychosocial measures are used to structure the environment for therapeutic ends (for example, provide for paternal participation in all phases of the maternity experience).
• Group behaviors are used to structure interaction and influence the therapeutic environment.
  Approaches are specified to orient the patient to:
• new roles and relationships
• relevant health resources, both human and material
• modifications in the plan of nursing care
• relation of modifications in nursing care plan to the total care plan.
  The plan of nursing care includes the utilization of available and appropriate resources, including:
• human resources, such as other health care personnel
• material resources
• community resources.
  The plan includes an ordered sequence of nursing actions.
  Nursing approaches are planned on the basis of current scientific knowledge.

### Standard V

Nursing actions provide for patient participation in health promotion, maintenance, and restoration.

### Rationale
The patient and family are continually involved in nursing care.

### Assessment factors
The patient and family are kept informed about:
• current health status
• changes in health status
• total health care plan
• nursing care plan

(continued)

## A.N.A.'S STANDARDS OF NURSING PRACTICE *(continued)*

• roles of health care personnel
• health care resources.
   The patient and family are provided with the information needed to make decisions about:
• promoting, maintaining, and restoring health
• seeking and utilizing appropriate health care personnel
• maintaining and using health care resources.

### Standard VI

Nursing actions assist the patient to maximize his health capabilities.

#### Rationale
Nursing actions are designed to promote, maintain, and restore health.

#### Assessment factors
Nursing actions:
• are consistent with the plan of care
• are based on scientific principles
• are individualized to the specific situation
• are used to provide a safe and therapeutic environment
• use teaching and learning opportunities for the patient
• include utilization of appropriate resources.
   Nursing actions are guided by the patient's physical, physiologic, psychological, and social behavior associated with:
• ingestion of food, fluid, and nutrients
• elimination of body wastes and excesses in fluid
• locomotion and exercise
• regulatory mechanisms—body heat, metabolism
• relating to others
• self-actualization.

### Standard VII

The patient's progress or lack of progress toward goal achievement is determined by the patient and the nurse.

#### Rationale
The quality of nursing care depends on comprehensive and intelligent determination of nursing's impact on the patient's health status. The patient is an essential part of this determination.

#### Assessment factors
Current data about the patient are used to measure his progress toward goal achievement.
   Nursing actions are used for their effectiveness in helping the patient achieve goals.
   The patient evaluates nursing actions and goal achievement.
   Provision is made for follow-up to determine the long-term effects of nursing care on the patient.

### Standard VIII

The patient's progress or lack of progress toward goal achievement directs reassessment, reordering of priorities, setting new goals, and revising the plan of nursing care.

#### Rationale
The nursing process remains the same, but the input of new information may dictate new or revised approaches.

#### Assessment factors
Reassessment is directed by achievement or lack of goal achievement.
   New priorities and goals are determined and additional nursing approaches are prescribed appropriately.
   New nursing actions are accurately and appropriately initiated.

## N.A.N.D.A. TAXONOMY I REVISED

In 1986, the North American Nursing Diagnosis Association (NANDA) published its first list of nursing diagnoses, known as the NANDA Taxonomy I. In 1990, NANDA published the revised version shown here. As you'll see, the system is organized around nine human response patterns.

**Pattern 1. Exchanging: A human response pattern involving mutual giving and receiving**

| | |
|---|---|
| 1.1.2.1 | Altered nutrition: More than body requirements |
| 1.1.2.2 | Altered nutrition: Less than body requirements |
| 1.1.2.3 | Altered nutrition: Potential for more than body requirements |
| 1.2.1.1 | Potential for infection |
| 1.2.2.1 | Potential for altered body temperature |
| 1.2.2.2 | Hypothermia |
| 1.2.2.3 | Hyperthermia |
| 1.2.2.4 | Ineffective thermoregulation |
| 1.2.3.1 | Dysreflexia |
| 1.3.1.1 | Constipation |
| 1.3.1.1.1 | Perceived constipation |
| 1.3.1.1.2 | Colonic constipation |
| 1.3.1.2 | Diarrhea |
| 1.3.1.3 | Bowel incontinence |
| 1.3.2 | Altered urinary elimination |
| 1.3.2.1.1 | Stress incontinence |
| 1.3.2.1.2 | Reflex incontinence |
| 1.3.2.1.3 | Urge incontinence |
| 1.3.2.1.4 | Functional incontinence |
| 1.3.2.1.5 | Total incontinence |
| 1.3.2.2 | Urinary retention |
| 1.4.1.1 | Altered (specify type) tissue perfusion (renal, cerebral, cardiopulmonary, gastrointestinal, peripheral) |
| 1.4.1.2.1 | Fluid volume excess |
| 1.4.1.2.2.1 | Fluid volume deficit |
| 1.4.1.2.2.2 | Potential fluid volume deficit |
| 1.4.2.1 | Decreased cardiac output |
| 1.5.1.1 | Impaired gas exchange |
| 1.5.1.2 | Ineffective airway clearance |
| 1.5.1.3 | Ineffective breathing pattern |
| 1.6.1 | Potential for injury |
| 1.6.1.1 | Potential for suffocation |
| 1.6.1.2 | Potential for poisoning |
| 1.6.1.3 | Potential for trauma |
| 1.6.1.4 | Potential for aspiration |
| 1.6.1.5 | Potential for disuse syndrome |
| 1.6.2 | Altered protection |
| 1.6.2.1 | Impaired tissue integrity |
| 1.6.2.1.1 | Altered oral mucous membrane |
| 1.6.2.1.2.1 | Impaired skin integrity |
| 1.6.2.1.2.2 | Potential impaired skin integrity |

**Pattern 2. Communicating: A human response pattern involving sending messages**

| | |
|---|---|
| 2.1.1.1 | Impaired verbal communication |

**Pattern 3. Relating: A human response pattern involving establishing bonds**

| | |
|---|---|
| 3.1.1 | Impaired social interaction |
| 3.1.2 | Social isolation |
| 3.2.1 | Altered role performance |
| 3.2.1.1.1 | Altered parenting |
| 3.2.1.1.2 | Potential altered parenting |
| 3.2.1.2.1 | Sexual dysfunction |
| 3.2.2 | Altered family processes |
| 3.2.3.1 | Parental role conflict |
| 3.3 | Altered sexuality patterns |

**Pattern 4. Valuing: A human response pattern involving the assigning of relative worth**

| | |
|---|---|
| 4.1.1 | Spiritual distress (distress of the human spirit) |

**Pattern 5. Choosing: A human response pattern involving the selection of alternatives**

| | |
|---|---|
| 5.1.1.1 | Ineffective individual coping |
| 5.1.1.1.1 | Impaired adjustment |
| 5.1.1.1.2 | Defensive coping |
| 5.1.1.1.3 | Ineffective denial |
| 5.1.2.1.1 | Ineffective family coping: Disabling |
| 5.1.2.1.2 | Ineffective family coping: Compromised |
| 5.1.2.2 | Family coping: Potential for growth |
| 5.2.1.1 | Noncompliance (specify) |
| 5.3.1.1 | Decisional conflict (specify) |
| 5.4 | Health-seeking behaviors (specify) |

*(continued)*

## N.A.N.D.A. TAXONOMY I REVISED *(continued)*

**Pattern 6. Moving: A human response pattern involving activity**
| | |
|---|---|
| 6.1.1.1 | Impaired physical mobility |
| 6.1.1.2 | Activity intolerance |
| 6.1.1.2.1 | Fatigue |
| 6.1.1.3 | Potential activity intolerance |
| 6.2.1 | Sleep pattern disturbance |
| 6.3.1.1 | Diversional activity deficit |
| 6.4.1.1 | Impaired home maintenance management |
| 6.4.2 | Altered health maintenance |
| 6.5.1 | Feeding self-care deficit |
| 6.5.1.1 | Impaired swallowing |
| 6.5.1.2 | Ineffective breast-feeding |
| 6.5.1.3 | Effective breast-feeding |
| 6.5.2 | Bathing/hygiene self-care deficit |
| 6.5.3 | Dressing/grooming self-care deficit |
| 6.5.4 | Toileting self-care deficit |
| 6.6 | Altered growth and development |

**Pattern 7. Perceiving: A human response pattern involving the reception of information**
| | |
|---|---|
| 7.1.1 | Body image disturbance |
| 7.1.2 | Self-esteem disturbance |
| 7.1.2.1 | Chronic low self-esteem |
| 7.1.2.2 | Situational low self-esteem |
| 7.1.3 | Personal identity disturbance |
| 7.2 | Sensory/perceptual alterations (specify visual, auditory, kinesthetic, gustatory, tactile, olfactory) |
| 7.2.1.1 | Unilateral neglect |
| 7.3.1 | Hopelessness |
| 7.3.2 | Powerlessness |

**Pattern 8. Knowing: A human response pattern involving the meaning associated with information**
| | |
|---|---|
| 8.1.1 | Knowledge deficit (specify) |
| 8.3 | Altered thought processes |

**Pattern 9. Feeling: A human response pattern involving the subjective awareness of information**
| | |
|---|---|
| 9.1.1 | Pain |
| 9.1.1.1 | Chronic pain |
| 9.2.1.1 | Dysfunctional grieving |
| 9.2.1.2 | Anticipatory grieving |
| 9.2.2 | Potential for violence: Self-directed or directed at others |
| 9.2.3 | Posttrauma response |
| 9.2.3.1 | Rape-trauma syndrome |
| 9.2.3.1.1 | Rape-trauma syndrome: Compound reaction |
| 9.2.3.1.2 | Rape-trauma syndrome: Silent reaction |
| 9.3.1 | Anxiety |
| 9.3.2 | Fear |

# NURSING DIAGNOSES BASED ON GORDON'S SYSTEM

Marjory Gordon has developed a system of functional health patterns, which you can use to organize the information you gather during your initial assessment and to group your nursing diagnoses. Below you'll find a listing of Gordon's functional health patterns along with their corresponding nursing diagnoses.

**1. Health perception and health management pattern**
- Altered protection
- Disuse syndrome, potential
- Dysreflexia
- Health maintenance alteration
- Health-seeking behaviors
- Infection, potential
- Injury, potential
- Noncompliance
- Poisoning, potential
- Suffocation, potential

**2. Nutritional and metabolic pattern**
- Body temperature alteration, potential
- Breast-feeding, effective
- Breast-feeding, ineffective
- Fluid volume deficit
- Fluid volume deficit, potential
- Fluid volume excess
- Hyperthermia
- Hypothermia
- Nutrition alteration: Less than body requirements
- Nutrition alteration: More than body requirements
- Nutrition alteration: Potential for more than body requirements
- Oral mucous membrane alteration
- Skin integrity impairment
- Skin integrity impairment, potential
- Swallowing impairment
- Thermoregulation, ineffective
- Tissue integrity impairment

**3. Elimination pattern**
- Constipation
- Diarrhea
- Incontinence, bowel

- Incontinence, functional
- Incontinence, reflex
- Incontinence, stress
- Incontinence, total
- Incontinence, urge
- Urinary elimination pattern alteration
- Urinary retention

**4. Activity or exercise pattern**
- Activity intolerance
- Activity intolerance, potential
- Airway clearance, ineffective
- Aspiration, potential
- Breathing pattern, ineffective
- Cardiac output decrease
- Diversional activity deficit
- Gas exchange impairment
- Impaired home maintenance management
- Mobility impairment
- Neglect, unilateral
- Self-care deficit
- Tissue perfusion alteration

**5. Sleep and rest pattern**
- Fatigue
- Sleep pattern disturbance

**6. Cognitive and perceptual pattern**
- Knowledge deficit
- Pain
- Pain, chronic
- Sensory-perceptual alteration
- Thought process impairment

**7. Self-perception and self-concept pattern**
- Adjustment impairment
- Anxiety
- Body image disturbance
- Fear
- Hopelessness

- Personal identity disturbance
- Powerlessness
- Self-esteem, chronic low
- Self-esteem, situational low
- Self-esteem disturbance
- Violence, potential

**8. Role or relationship pattern**
- Family process alteration
- Grieving, anticipatory
- Grieving, dysfunctional
- Parental role conflict
- Parenting, alteration: Actual or potential
- Social interaction impairment
- Social isolation
- Verbal communication impairment
- Violence, potential

**9. Sexuality and reproductive pattern**
- Rape-trauma syndrome
- Sexual dysfunction
- Sexual pattern alteration

**10. Coping and stress-tolerance pattern**
- Coping, defensive
- Coping, family
- Coping, ineffective family
- Coping, ineffective individual
- Decisional conflict
- Denial
- Grieving, dysfunctional
- Growth and development alteration

**11. Value and belief pattern**
- Spiritual distress

# NURSING DIAGNOSES BASED ON OREM'S THEORY

Dorothea Orem's theory of nursing emphasizes self-care activities that maintain life, health, and well-being. The list below contains Orem's universal self-care requirements and their related nursing diagnoses.

## Air
- Airway clearance, ineffective
- Aspiration, potential
- Breathing pattern, ineffective
- Gas exchange, impaired

## Water
- Cardiac output, decreased
- Fluid volume deficit
- Fluid volume deficit, potential
- Fluid volume excess
- Tissue perfusion alteration

## Food
- Breast-feeding, effective
- Breast-feeding, ineffective
- Nutrition alteration: Less than body requirements
- Nutrition alteration: More than body requirements
- Nutrition alteration: Potential for more than body requirements
- Oral mucous membrane alteration

## Elimination
- Constipation
- Constipation, colonic
- Constipation, perceived
- Diarrhea
- Incontinence, bowel
- Incontinence, functional
- Incontinence, reflex
- Incontinence, stress
- Incontinence, total
- Incontinence, urge
- Skin integrity impairment
- Skin integrity impairment, potential
- Urinary elimination pattern alteration
- Urinary retention

## Activity and rest
- Activity intolerance
- Activity intolerance, potential
- Disuse syndrome, potential
- Diversional activity deficit
- Fatigue
- Mobility impairment
- Neglect, unilateral
- Self-care deficit
- Sleep pattern disturbance

## Solitude and social interaction
- Family process alteration
- Parental role conflict
- Parenting alteration, actual or potential
- Rape-trauma syndrome
- Role performance alteration
- Sexual dysfunction
- Sexuality pattern alteration
- Social interaction impairment
- Social isolation
- Verbal communication impairment
- Violence, potential: Self-directed or directed at others

## Prevention of hazards
- Altered protection
- Body temperature alteration, potential
- Dysreflexia
- Health maintenance alteration
- Health-seeking behaviors
- Home maintenance management impairment
- Hyperthermia
- Hypothermia
- Infection, potential
- Injury, potential

- Noncompliance
- Pain
- Pain, chronic
- Poisoning, potential
- Suffocation, potential
- Swallowing impairment
- Thermoregulation, ineffective
- Tissue integrity impairment
- Trauma, potential

## Promotion of human functioning
- Adjustment impairment
- Anxiety
- Body image disturbance
- Coping, defensive
- Coping, ineffective family
- Coping, ineffective individual
- Decisional conflict
- Denial
- Family coping: Potential for growth
- Fear
- Grieving, anticipatory
- Grieving, dysfunctional
- Growth and development alteration
- Hopelessness
- Knowledge deficit
- Personal identity disturbance
- Posttrauma response
- Powerlessness
- Self-esteem, chronic low
- Self-esteem, situational low
- Self-esteem disturbance
- Sensory-perceptual alteration
- Spiritual distress
- Thought process alteration

# COMPARING NURSING THEORIES

Nursing theories differ in their assumptions about patients and health, the goals of nursing, and research and practice methods. Each theory usually includes a definition of nursing, a statement of purpose, and definitions of person, health, and environment. The chart below gives you a quick overview of eight theories.

| DEFINITION OF NURSING | PURPOSE OF NURSING | DEFINITION OF PERSON, HEALTH, AND ENVIRONMENT |
| --- | --- | --- |
| **Nightingale's model** | | |
| • A profession for women that seeks to discover and use nature's laws governing health to serve humanity | • To put the person in the best condition for nature to restore or preserve health<br>• To prevent or cure disease and injury | *Person*<br>• A being composed of physical, intellectual, and metaphysical attributes and potentials<br>*Health*<br>• To be free of disease and able to use one's own powers to the fullest<br>*Environment*<br>• External elements that affect the healthy or sick person |
| **Henderson's model** | | |
| • A profession that assists the individual, sick or well, in activities contributing to health or recovery | • To carry out 14 components of nursing care | *Person*<br>• A biological being with inseparable mind and body<br>*Health*<br>• To be able to function independently (using the 14 components of nursing care as a guide)<br>*Environment*<br>• Not clearly defined, but can act on a person in a positive or negative way |
| **Levine's model** | | |
| • A human interaction incorporating scientific principles into the nursing process | • To provide individualized holistic care<br>• To support each person's adaptations | *Person*<br>• A complex individual who interacts with internal and external environments and adapts to change<br>*Health*<br>• A pattern of adaptive change<br>• To be whole<br>*Environment*<br>• Internally, the person's physiology<br>• Externally, the perceptual, operational, and conceptual components |

*(continued)*

## COMPARING NURSING THEORIES *(continued)*

| DEFINITION OF NURSING | PURPOSE OF NURSING | DEFINITION OF PERSON, HEALTH, AND ENVIRONMENT |
|---|---|---|
| **Orem's model** | | |
| • A human service designed to overcome limitations in health-related self-care | • To make judgments responding to a person's need for self-care to sustain life and health | *Person*<br>• An integral whole that functions biologically, symbolically, and socially<br>*Health*<br>• A state of wholeness or integrity of the individual, his or her parts, and modes of functioning<br>*Environment*<br>• A subcomponent of the person; together, they compose an integrated system related to self-care |
| **Roy's model** | | |
| • Analysis and action related to the care of an ill or potentially ill person | • To manipulate stimuli within a prescribed process of nursing assessment and intervention | *Person*<br>• A biopsychosocial being in constant interaction with a changing environment<br>• An open, adaptive system<br>*Health*<br>• Part of the health-illness continuum, a continuous line representing states or degrees of health or illness that a person might experience at a given time<br>*Environment*<br>• All conditions, circumstances, and influences surrounding and affecting the development of an organism or group of organisms |
| **Neuman's model** | | |
| • A profession concerned with the variables that affect the person's response to stressors | • To reduce a person's encounter with stressors<br>• To mitigate the effect of stressors | *Person*<br>• A physiologic, psychological, sociocultural, and developmental being<br>• Must be viewed as a whole<br>*Health*<br>• A state of wellness or illness determined by physiologic, psychological, sociocultural, and developmental variables that are relative and in a state of flux<br>*Environment*<br>• Internally, the state of the person in terms of physiologic, psychological, sociocultural, and developmental variables<br>• Externally, all that exists outside the person |

## COMPARING NURSING THEORIES *(continued)*

| DEFINITION OF NURSING | PURPOSE OF NURSING | DEFINITION OF PERSON, HEALTH, AND ENVIRONMENT |
|---|---|---|
| **King's model** | | |
| • Human interaction between nurse and client | • To exchange information with the patient and take action together to attain mutually set goals | *Person*<br>• An open system with permeable boundaries that permit the exchange of matter, energy, and information with the environment<br>*Health*<br>• Dynamic adjustment to stressors in the internal and external environment<br>• Makes optimal use of resources to achieve maximum potential for daily living<br>*Environment*<br>• An open system with permeable boundaries that permit the exchange of matter, energy, and information with human beings |
| **Rogers' model** | | |
| • A learned profession that promotes and maintains health and cares for and rehabilitates the sick and disabled | • To promote harmonious interaction between the environment and person | *Person*<br>• A four-dimensional energy field identified by pattern and organization and manifesting characteristics and behaviors that differ from those of its parts and that can't be predicted from knowledge of the parts<br>*Health*<br>• A value word broadly defined by cultures and individuals to describe behaviors considered to be of high or low value<br>*Environment*<br>• A four-dimensional energy field identified by pattern and organization and encompassing all that exists outside any given human field |

# INDEX

*t* refers to a table.

Joint Commission on Accreditation of
    Healthcare Organizations
  documentation standards of, 29, 169
  requirements of, for patient assessment,
      70-72
Judgmental statements, avoidance of, 33

**KL**
Kardex, 23
  cover sheet for, 24-25
King's theory, 179t
Learning needs of patient, documenting,
    77
Learning outcomes, 108, 110
  writing, 108-109
Legal documents, witnessing signature
    on, 48, 52
Legal protection, clinical record as, 5
Levine's theory, 177t
Licensing of health care facility, 2-3
Living wills, 53, 54

**M**
Malpractice
  causes of lawsuits for, 40
  documentation and, 39-41
  elements of, 39, 41
Managed care, 115. *See also* Case man-
    agement.
Maslow's hierarchy of needs, 93, 94
Medication administration, documenting,
    128, 130

**N**
NANDA. *See* North American Nursing Di-
    agnosis Association taxonomy I Re-
    vised.
Narrative documentation, 14, 16, 130,
    131, 132, 133
  advantages and disadvantages of, 133
  for initial assessment, 72
Neuman's theory, 178t
Nightingale's theory, 177t
North American Nursing Diagnosis Asso-
    ciation taxonomy I Revised, 173-174
Nurses' notes, signing, 33, 35, 37
Nursing assessment, medical model for,
    74, 75-76, 77
Nursing care plan. *See* Care plans,
    nursing.

Nursing diagnoses
  assessment data as basis for, 92
  based on Gordon's system, 175
  based on Orem's theory, 176
  components of, 91-93
  documenting, 11
  formulating, 11, 90-93
    guidelines for, 91
  NANDA taxonomy I Revised, 173-174
Nursing information systems, computer-
    ized documentation and, 19
Nursing minimum data set, computerized
    documentation and, 19-21
Nursing process, documentation and,
    9-13
Nursing theories, comparison of, 177-179t

**O**
Objective charting, 33, 34
Objective data, 62
Omissions, charting of, 39
Ongoing assessment, 83-85
  documenting, 85
Open-ended form for initial assessment,
    72, 73
Orem's theory, 178t
  nursing diagnoses based on, 176
Outcome statements
  components of, 95
  writing, 95-97

**P**
Patient consent, 43-44
Patient discharge, documenting, 148-149,
    150
Patient interview, 63-64, 67-68
  creating setting for, 66-67
  timesaving measures for, 68, 69
Patient outcome, 93
Patient privacy, 55-57
Patient responses, charting, 123
Patient teaching
  benefits of, 145-146
  documenting, 145-150
  using narrative notes, 146-147
Patient-teaching plan, 102, 107-108, 110,
    113. *See also* Patient teaching.
  components of, 107-108, 110
  content of, 110
  documenting, 113
  flow sheet for, 114
  learning needs and, 108

*t* refers to a table.